Health Care Without Shame

A Handbook
for the Sexually Diverse
and Their Caregivers

by Charles Moser, Ph.D., M.D.

greenery
press

Published in the United States by Greenery Press, 3739 Balboa Ave. PMB 195, San Francisco, CA 94121.

http://www.bigrock.com/~greenery

ISBN 0-890159-12-3

Contents

Foreword, by Eli Coleman, Ph.D. .... *iv*

Part One: For Consumers

Introduction 3

Some Background 11

Portrait of a Sex-Positive Health Care Practitioner 17

"Doc, There's Something I Want to Tell You..." 33

Being a Savvy Patient 49

How Can You Tell If It's Working? 55

When It Goes Wrong 59

What If Your Practitioner Isn't Available? 67

Working With Other Professionals 77

Part Two: For Practitioners

Some Background for the Practitioner 89

A Brief Overview of Sexual Minorities & Health Issues 99

Part Three: Conclusion and Resource Guide

Conclusion 113

Resource Guide 117

Other Books by Greenery Press 122

Whether you are someone searching for a sensitive, non-judgmental doctor to treat you with respect and dignity or you are a health care provider trying to learn how to treat your sexually diverse patient population with a professional attitude and concern, this book is enormously helpful.

As a professor of family medicine and director of the Program in Human Sexuality at the University of Minnesota's Medical School, I am the course director of our human sexuality course for medical students. I have been teaching them for over twenty years. I know that while some students never want to know or understand the diversity of human sexuality expression, most of the students are deeply concerned about how they will better approach their patients in a professional manner. Most want to be careful not to impose their own values or experiences on their patients. They realize that the world is very diverse and that they will encounter many individuals with sexualities different from their own. They are eager to better understand what people do sexually and to develop some understanding of their path in life. Not all medical schools are like ours, but I see positive changes everywhere.

It seems that more and more physicians want to approach their patients in this manner. Perhaps this is driven by a greater realization in society of the great diversity of human sexuality and how we have unnecessarily pathologized this diversity in the past. I think it is also driven by a greater openness within the medical profession to express sexual diversity among themselves. For example, many years ago, I so clearly remember how painful it was for gay and lesbian medical students to go through their medical training in absolute secrecy. Now, if you are gay or lesbian, you don't have to hide that anymore. There is much greater openness. For example, there are gay and lesbian medical associations in most medical schools today.

In any event, individuals with diverse sexual behaviors, practices, and identities are more likely to find physicians who are ready to provide high quality medical care in a professional manner. That is not to say that all physicians are like that. And that is why the helpful suggestions that Dr. Moser gives you in this book will help you find those individuals and work with those who might not completely understand your behavior or identity. No one will get medical care today if s/he is not assertive and willing to participate in treatment. And understandably, "coming out" is not always an easy thing, especially if you are still exploring and trying to understand your sexuality yourself. But, seeing a physician and talking openly about your sexual behavior practices and identity is an opportunity to explore being yourself and get comfortable with yourself.

Unnecessary guilt and shame about your sexuality are bad for your health. They can create anxiety, depression, substance abuse and dependency. And most of all, guilt and shame rob you of the joy of life and the ability to enjoy one of life's greatest gifts – your sexuality. Search for peace, harmony, and health with your sexuality. Some behaviors are just plain unhealthy but most problems come from the guilt and shame that are associated with them. If you are unsure or uncomfortable with your sexuality, there are sensitive health care professionals who are out there who can assist you.

Remember that physicians are, above all, healers. They take an oath: "Do no harm." Going to a physician is a place to heal. So with the right attitude of both the patient and physician, amazing things can happen. Certainly, there is nothing more valued by most people than having an "askable physician" – one you can talk about anything with and you know will simply give reasoned help and advice based upon science rather than morality.

Dr. Moser is a role model for all health care providers. They can certainly benefit from his advice. Expect nothing less from your physician or other health care providers and we will all learn to live together – respecting and helping one another and creating a sexually healthier society.

Eli Coleman, Ph.D.
Professor and Director, Program in Human Sexuality, Department of Family Practice and Community Health, University of Minnesota Medical School

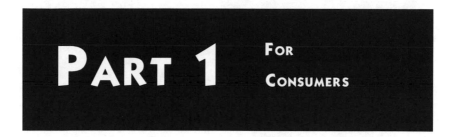

PART 1 FOR CONSUMERS

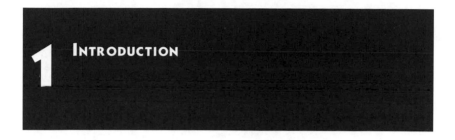

1 INTRODUCTION

Some years ago, a man came to me as a first-time patient, saying he'd picked me as his primary care physician because of my open attitude about alternative sexual behaviors and lifestyles. During his history and physical, he told me he was monogamous and heterosexual. He denied engaging in any alternative sexual behaviors himself. When I asked about the scars on his abdomen, he told me they were from an emergency appendectomy.

Thus, a few months later when he showed up in the emergency room with a high fever, complaining of right lower quadrant abdominal pain, looking and sounding like someone with acute appendicitis, I was stumped. Instead of rushing him off to surgery, I was getting ready to order some very expensive tests. Then one of the nurses in the ER recognized him – she'd worked in his previous doctor's office. "I don't know about an appendectomy," she told me, "but at least one of those scars is from where we did surgery to take out the dildo he had lodged in his colon." We were able to rush him to the operating room and do the appendectomy he needed – but by concealing his sexual practices from me, he'd endangered his own life.

It's stories like this one that inspired me to write this book. As one of a handful of openly sex- and kink-positive physicians in the U.S., I hear such sad tales almost daily – in person, by phone and mail, on the Internet, and at "Ask The Doctor" speaking engagements. Many people with unusual sexual lifestyles do not dare tell their physicians about their problems, too often with tragic consequences.

My concern about such people was a major factor in my choice to become a doctor in the first place. Today, I have a private practice in San Francisco focusing on the medical aspects of sexual problems and the sexual aspects of medical problems. The care of sexual minorities (by which I mean anyone who is not traditionally heterosexual) is a large part of my practice.

When I was in training to be an internist (a specialist in adult medicine), a very respected and popular physician, one of my teachers, took me aside for some fatherly advice. He put his arm around my shoulder and had a heart-to-heart talk with me. He told me I was a good doctor and *could* be very successful, but to forget about this sex stuff; it would hurt my credibility as a doctor. If I had taken his advice, I might have been asked to join his large and prestigious practice. Needless to say, I rejected it. (I wonder what he'll think when he sees this book!) I still get this physician's personal patients seeking me out for care of their sexual issues. And he still insists that he never sees sexually unusual patients in his practice.

Yet this doctor's approach to sexuality is the rule, not the exception: The medical profession is not generally very understanding when it comes to sexual issues, and lacks the researach foundation upon which other aspects of medicine are based. One of my medical school professors taught that the first touch of a pelvic exam should not be to the woman's genitals, because such a touch might be interpreted as an assault. Instead, I was told, I should touch her knee first, then lightly run my gloved hand down her thigh to her genitals. Another professor said that the thigh is an erogenous zone and that touching a woman there was very erotic, and thus inappropriate. This kind of schizophrenia is unfortunately typical of medical training regarding sexuality – confusing doctors, often into inaction.

My medical school offered just one lecture on examining patients with sexual concerns; it was taught by a nurse-practitioner. While nurse-practitioners are an integral part of the health care team, the only time they ordinarily teach classes to medical students is when a subject comes up that the physicians decline to teach (a distinction which is not lost on the medical students). During the lecture, a young well-built male medical student asked what to do if a male patient gets an erection during the exam – cover it with a towel, leave the room, or ignore it and proceed with the examination? The nurse practitioner ignored the question, and the student (not me!) persistently kept asking. We never got an answer. And that was the sum total of my medical school education on sexuality.

The sad truth is that many people with unusual sexual lifestyles and behaviors – including gays, lesbians and bisexuals, folks who enjoy S/M, who have body modifications such as piercings or tattoos, who crossdress, who are sex workers, who have multiple partners, who are transgendered, who engage in fetish behaviors – are not getting the health care *they need and deserve.* For some, of course, the problem is financial: many such folk are too far out of the mainstream; they lack conventional jobs that offer medical insurance and cannot afford to buy their own. And many more are fearful of being judged, lectured to, mistreated – or perhaps even reported to their employers, their spouses or the police – if they seek medical help for even the most ordinary of complaints. Simple problems fester until they become chronic, serious, or even life-threatening.

Perhaps even more worrisome is such folks' extension of their distrust of the practitioner to the entire science of medicine. Some of the people I meet have spent a small fortune on herbal remedies without much improvement, but still refuse to see a mainstream physician. While I'd be the last one to trash alternative medicine, I find it unfortunate when anyone overlooks important potential treatments simply because they're administered by the medical establishment they distrust.

The present situation is unconscionable. People – gay or bi or straight, kinky or vanilla, celibate or sexually active, employed or un- – deserve competent, caring, nonjudgmental health care. Nobody should be harmed, suffer unnecessary pain or illness or injury, because their sexual behavior makes them too fearful or ashamed to seek treatment. It is well beyond the time for sexual minorities to demand respect and care from their physicians, chiropractors, therapists and other professionals.

When I decided to go to medical school, I had the same anti-physician bias: I believed that all physicians were conservative Republicans with moralizing attitudes. I remember giving myself pep talks to help me fit into the conservative aspects of medical school. I have learned that my original beliefs were, in many if not most cases, quite wrong. Through medical school and my subsequent private practice, I have been amazed at the number of physicians who will provide excellent medical care without judgments.

When I started my internal medicine practice, I became an associate with another physician also specializing in internal medicine. Like most internists, his practice was composed primarily of older patients, and the kind of folks who were coming to see me might be a shock to his office staff and to his patients. He did a wonderful job talking to his staff, explaining, "Our job is to take care of sick people; we don't care about anything else." He explained that the sickest patients should be seen first, and briefed the staff about how to deal with patients who have a hard time being appropriate in a doctor's office. My staff, the other physicians I work with, and the hospitals where I admit patients (including a Catholic hospital), have all been wonderfully accepting.

Nonetheless, there were problems. One of my associate's patients was sitting in the waiting room when an obviously transsexual patient of mine came in to see me. A couple of months later, my associate's patient had a stroke, and discovered when his family called that I was on call that weekend. He refused to go to the hospital, insisting that "Dr. Moser takes care of weird people." Finally, his daughter cajoled him into going, and I was able to take good care of him. Later, while he was recovering, he admitted to me that he felt foolish. "I thought you were such a bad doctor that people like that were the only patients you could get," he confessed. "Now I know that you're such a good doctor you'll take care of whoever needs you."

On a similar note, I've been surprised, and sometimes a little dismayed, at the number of members of the kink community who prejudge their physicians because of sex, religious affiliation, or the physician's own lifestyle choices.

This, then, is the goal of *Health Care Without Shame.* I hope that it will be read by two types of people – by people who want help in finding and/or opening up to professionals who will provide them with competent and nonjudgmental health care, and by those professionals who want to know more about sexual minorities so that they can render more effective care. I'd like to see us all on the same side, working together toward a mutual goal of better health care for everyone.

Unfortunately, most professionals have had little or no training in human sexuality. They may never have knowingly met anyone kinky. Unless they take the initiative to seek out information on their own, they have been taught very little about alternative sexualities. They often do not understand the medical problems related to the practice of various sexual behaviors, nor the issues inherent in various sexual lifestyles.

Most have read few if any of the excellent books written by and for members of sexual minorities.

If you are a health care professional, I hope this book can give you some insight into understanding and communicating with your sexually active patients, especially those with alternative sexual lifestyles. This sensitivity and knowledge will enable you to treat all your patients in a more caring and effective manner.

If you identify as a sexual minority or engage in non-traditional sexual behaviors, I want to give you some ideas about how to find health care professionals who will be able to give you the care you deserve, and how to talk to them once you find them. In today's health care environment – where even the most caring of physicians has *at most* fifteen minutes to spend with each patient – it's important that you understand what kind of information your health care professional needs, and the best ways to present that information. (Remember, the only way he has of knowing whether you're a happy self-actualized pervert or a desperate abuse victim or a potential mental patient is the information you provide!) I also hope to give you some skills and suggestions regarding how to proceed if your physician is not accepting of your lifestyle.

So if you're a doctor, psychologist, chiropractor, osteopath, nurse, physician's assistant, therapist, physical therapist, dentist, massage therapist, or perhaps even an accountant or attorney...

Or you're a submissive, polyamorist, crossdresser, transgendered person, sex worker, asexual, sexual only with yourself, sadist, fetishist, dominant, intersexed, modern primitive, swinger, or perhaps even simply gay, lesbian or bisexual...

... please allow this book to act as an introduction.

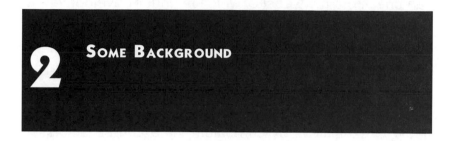

2 **Some Background**

On me. So who am I and what entitles me to write this book?

My primary interest for most of my adult life has been the scientific study of sexuality (sexology). I have made my living as a clinical sexologist (sex therapist) and now as a physician. I received a MSW (master's degree in social work) from the University of Washington in Seattle, and am an LCSW (Licensed Clinical Social Worker) in California. I earned my Ph.D. from the Institute for Advanced Study in Human Sexuality in 1979, after which I was invited to be on their faculty. I am now a Professor of Sexology and Dean of Professional Studies there. I went on to earn my M.D. degree from Hahnemann University School of Medicine in Philadelphia in 1991. I am board-certified in Internal Medicine and am also a board-certified Sexologist. I maintain a private internal medicine practice in San Francisco, with a focus on sexual concerns and the medical problems of sexual minorities.

In addition to my work, I have served as the President of the Western Region of the Society of Scientific Study of Sexuality and am on the Editorial Board of *San Francisco Medicine*. I am in the process of forming the American College of Sexual Medicine and Health, an organization of physicians interested in the sexual aspects of medicine. (You can check out my website, which is under development at this time, at http://pweb.netcom.com/~docx2/ACSMH.html). I have published numerous academic papers on sexual topics, including nipple piercing, sadomasochism, safer sex, orgasm, and the effects of recreational drugs on sexual functioning. In addition, I am a frequent speaker and expert witness on alternative sexualities. My curriculum vitae can be accessed on-line at http://pweb.netcom.com/~docx2/cv.html.

On the terminology in this book. The increasing complexity of today's health care system has made some of the terminology in this book rather challenging. It is no longer realistic to assume that the first or only health care practitioner a patient is likely to see will be a doctor of medicine (M.D.) – it might just as well be a doctor of chiropractic, an osteopath, a nurse, nurse practitioner or physician's assistant, or a naturopath.

Happily, we can also no longer assume that the health care practitioner in question will be male.

Therefore, throughout this book, I have alternated between "he" and "she" in discussing both health care practitioners and their patients. And, while I will sometimes refer to the health care practitioner as a "physician" for reasons of brevity, I hope you will understand that the suggestions

I make will apply equally to whomever your health caregiver might be.

I've also done my best to define my terms as I go regarding sexual identities and behaviors, but the fast-changing nature of cultural perceptions of sexuality has made this difficult. Chapter Eleven of this book includes a glossary for further clarification.

On the health care system. For you to understand many of the ideas in this book, you need a little bit of background on the realities of today's health care system. Medicine has become very large, very complex, and very much a business.

Many people today belong to health care maintenance organizations (HMOs), which provide care for a lower monthly premium than other forms of health coverage. HMOs operate by paying each physician a monthly fee for each patient who chooses him as a primary care physician. Physicians join an independent practice association (IPA). The HMO makes a deal with the IPA, often without consulting either the patients or the physicians who have to live with the results. As a general rule, you pay for what you get.

The HMO's goal is to enroll patients who will pay their fees while utilizing as few of their resources as possible. The physicians' goal is to enroll so many healthy patients – who rarely if ever need to see a doctor – that they can make enough money to give their sick patients all the time they need.

In this style of managed care, enrolling as many patients as possible is the only way to make money. The larger the number of people on your "panel" (patients signed up with you), the more money you make. By signing up a patient, the physician takes on the responsibility of caring for that patient. Since there are only so many hours in the day, seeing patients efficiently and quickly is the key.

Obviously, then, there is an economic disadvantage to being known as an expert in treating patients with high-maintenance conditions. While it is unethical (and rare) for a physician to refuse to see sick patients, some physicians do apply subtle pressures to convince a sick patient to change physicians. Therefore, some of the advice you will read in this book is designed to help you present yourself to your health care practitioner as someone who will probably not be an exceptionally demanding patient.

Clinics and government-supported care. Many people with alternative sexualities have lifestyles that do not permit them to obtain private health care, even through an HMO. If you are such a person, you may be getting your medical care in a clinic, or through a government-supported program such as Medicaid.

Free clinics are usually supported by various charities and/or religious groups. They usually have a mission: the homeless, the working poor, women, drug addicts, etc. These clinics are usually understanding about everyone's blemishes and are accustomed to seeing sexual minorities. They are usually quite tolerant, because they want the target group to use the clinic. Even the religious groups are fairly tolerant, sometimes even very tolerant.

Public clinics are supported by your tax dollars and also try to reach out to underserved groups. As with free clinics, they do not want to alienate their potential clientele, so they also tend to be fairly nonjudgmental. Sometimes you may get the feeling that they have a holier-than-thou attitude, but you will still get good care. A special type of public clinic is the STD (Sexually Transmitted Disease) Clinic. Their real purpose is to prevent the spread of STDs; therefore, they may take a dim view of non-monogamous sex, especially unprotected non-monogamous sex. Nevertheless, they will give you good care.

Planned Parenthood and similar clinics provide medical and reproductive care, primarily to women. They are supported by a variety of grants, fees, and other sources of income.

Medicare is a federal program which provides medical care (but not prescriptions or long-term care) for the aged and permanently disabled.

Medicaid (MediCal in California) is a health insurance program for indigent people (people on general assistance, and, in some states, the "working poor"). It is a government program, run by the states with mostly federal money. It pays its providers rather badly, so many doctors limit the number of Medicaid patients that they accept. For some people, it is combined with Medicare.

Institutional care. If you are in prison or the armed forces, you have even more problems to solve: these are places where the administration might not care that you are upset with your medical care. Good interpersonal skills can take you a long way, but the world is not perfect. Depending on the situation, it may be better for you to lie about or deny your sexual interests. Hopefully, as medicine becomes more aware of these issues, it will filter down into even the darkest corners of prejudice. Meanwhile, however, there are many enlightened physicians working in these settings.

Outside the U.S. If you live outside the U.S., you probably live under some form of government-managed health care program. Some of the notes above, and further on in this book, can help you understand a bit more about how your health care system works and how to get the most from it. I cannot go into details about the health care system in every country; foreign countries differ greatly in both culture and the way they administer medical care. If you can find other practitioners of your lifestyle where you live, it may help to see how they have solved the problem. You may be able to ascertain what approaches have either worked or not worked for them. It may also help to find one or more physicians who practice in your culture, who may be able to give you insights as to how to approach your medical system.

The purpose of this long-winded section is to explain (but not defend) why it sometimes seems that your physician is rushing through the appointment. It may also help you understand some of the pressures on your physician.

With a clearer understanding of the context in which most people these days receive their health care, let's move on to finding out more about how sexual minorities can get the health care they need.

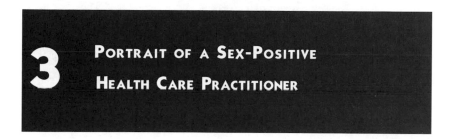

3 PORTRAIT OF A SEX-POSITIVE HEALTH CARE PRACTITIONER

So – you're looking for a lesbian internist with special expertise in anal fisting (or a gay ear-nose-and-throat doc who's not freaked out by your nineteen facial piercings, or a het female chiropractor who compliments your hummingbird tattoo with every thrust, or whatever).

Or are you?

Is it really critical that you find a practitioner who's a close match for you in terms of gender, age, sexual orientation, politics or religion? Or is it more important to find someone who's nonjudgmental about your various sexual practices and your lifestyle? How about someone who knows a lot about sex and associated problems, who's a good listener and who's willing to learn more about anything she doesn't already know about? Or how about a nice doctor, who will squeeze you in when it's really important, who teaches you something at every visit, who always seems to know the newest medical stuff that just hit the Internet last night? Remember, you're looking for medical care, not a life partner.

I've seen sexual minority patients pass up excellent, nonjudgmental physicians for all the wrong reasons. During medical school, I did a stint working in a clinic under the supervision of a yarmulke-clad orthodox Jewish physician. I, and many of his prospective patients, assumed that he would be very conservative on sexual matters. In fact, he turned out to be extremely open-minded and a highly skilled physician – yet I saw members of sexual minorities flatly refuse to see him because they assumed that he would be judgmental, or that *they* just wouldn't feel comfortable. It was their loss.

You don't want to be judged by your gender, age, orientation, the way you dress or the way you look, and rightfully so. So why judge others the same way? It's good – not just ethically, but from a standpoint of getting the best possible health care – to give your potential practitioner the same break you ask for yourself.

Yet, clearly, not every health care practitioner is going to be a good choice for you. So in the absence of external cues such as gender or style of dress, how can you choose someone who will take good care of you *and* your sexuality?

What do you want? A good place to begin is by determining exactly what you want from your health care practitioner. We'd all love to be surrounded by people who think what we do is fabulous, who will never lecture us or disagree with us, and who will never act shocked or uncomfortable no matter how outrageous we are. This is probably neither a worthwhile nor an achievable goal.

There are important differences among physicians. Some are more aggressive in treating certain problems. Some emphasize lifestyle changes while others emphasize medication. Some do more preventive medicine than others. Personalities are different, some more formal, others more personal. Finding someone who is a good match for you in these qualities can be just as important as finding someone open to your sexual lifestyle and behaviors.

Let's keep in mind here that the number-one quality you want in someone who will be taking care of your health is *competence*. The vast majority of physicians know the basics of medicine and when they need to refer patients to another doctor because a problem is outside their own expertise. Competence is that, and much more. It is the ability to listen to you attentively and respectfully. It is also the ability to impart information in a way you can hear it, answer your questions, and invoke a sense of trust. If you actually trust what she says and make a good-faith effort to follow her instructions, so much the better. If you feel that you can go back to her when the first intervention didn't work to make a second attempt, that's better yet.

It doesn't matter how friendly and nonjudgmental she is, if she's a bad doctor. Remember, this isn't just someone who writes out your antibiotic prescription when you have a bladder infection or gonorrhea; it's the person who will act as your intermediary with the entire health care world if anything serious ever happens to you. If you are unfortunate enough to be admitted to a hospital, you can't get a drink of water or an aspirin without your doctor's permission. She is the person who picks your surgeon, gastroenterologist and other specialists. If you're treated rudely by a nurse or lab tech, she's the one who has the best shot at making sure it never happens again. And, most importantly, it's your physician who knows to try the newer and less invasive procedure, or to bypass it since you don't fit the criteria. Your physician is your advocate in the entire system.

You need someone whose expertise, discretion and professionalism you can trust absolutely – and if your choice comes down to a very good practitioner who frowns a bit when she hears that you're into play piercing, versus someone of questionable competence who thinks you're absolutely perfect just the way you are, I'd strongly recommend that you choose the first.

Some typical reactions. Some practitioners, if they find out that you are involved in an alternative sexual behavior or lifestyle, will react very negatively. In a worst-case scenario, they may refuse to treat you unless you quit engaging in whatever sexual practice it is that bothers them. (This is pretty rare.) They may have trouble believing that your choice to engage in alternative sexual behaviors is rational, unforced, and mentally healthy. They may ask questions ("*How* many people did you have sex with?!") or make statements that will lead you to believe that, even if they don't say so, they're deeply uncomfortable or judgmental about your personal sexual choices. It's probably best to steer clear of these.

Others will be a little bit uncomfortable or shocked. They may even lecture you a bit. But they will give you their very best health care regardless of what you like to do in the bedroom. This may be about the best you can do, particularly if you live in a small community. On the other hand, you're not planning on marrying this person – all you want is to get healthy and stay that way. Do you really need approval from your health care practitioner, or do you need competent and professional care?

Sometimes I refer patients to a specialist who I know is uncomfortable with alternative sexualities. I warn the patient, but I also explain that it's important to get the best medical opinion possible. I also take the situation as an opportunity to educate the specialist, preparing him by explaining the kink before he sees the patient and educating him afterwards. Knowing and interacting with a real person who engages in an alternative sexual lifestyle or behavior is very different than relating to a psychiatric diagnosis about which he's only read. The experience has made a noticeable difference in many of these specialists' acceptance levels.

Then there's the practitioner who may not have worked a lot with sexual minorities in the past, but is open-minded and willing to learn about alternative sexual behaviors. If someone is willing to admit what he doesn't know, that's always a good sign – as long as he's willing to spend some time learning.

Do not infer that just because Doctor X is personally involved in a particular alternative sexual behavior, he is knowledgeable about that behavior or about other types of sexual behaviors. Maintaining that level of expertise represents a major effort in terms of time and energy spent in research, in addition to the huge amount of time required simply to keep up with one's own specialty. Relatively few practitioners make the additional effort. Busy practitioners probably don't have the time to research your sexual practices as thoroughly as you would like. However, **it's *not* your job to educate this practitioner**; the information he needs is available from other sources besides you, and it's part of his job to find and learn what he needs to know. If he wants to learn more, steer him toward the information listed in the Resource Guide of this book.

When I was a resident, on a dermatology rotation, the dermatologist had a run-in with a gay male patient. I stepped in and cooled off the situation. Afterwards, this dermatologist complimented the way I handled the situation, which was my opening for some education. One of his comments was very revealing. He said, "I get along so well with the elderly women in my practice; I just don't know what I am doing wrong with the gay men." He recognized the problem without my pointing it out to him – he knew *something* was wrong, he just didn't know what. I knew this dermatologist and I knew he was not homophobic, but his style of interacting with elderly women came across as demeaning when translated to gay men. It was clear that he had thought about it and was frustrated with his lack of success. Don't assume that your physician doesn't want to do better.

Sexual minority subcultures often have very involved social structures. It is very easy for even a knowledgeable physician to make a *faux pas*, so a less experienced practitioner will almost certainly misspeak. Do not reject a physician because she does not understand the nuances of your sexual minority community – it is more important that you get competent medical care.

And finally, there's the handful of health care practitioners who make a special point of maintaining a high level of knowledge regarding alternative sexual behaviors. A sex-positive and sexually aware physician will be proactive in seeking out information about your sexual practices, and will not make assumptions about your sexuality based on your appearance or background. For example, if you identify as a lesbian, he will neither assume that you need birth control nor assume that you don't. His paperwork will reflect sexual realities regarding gender (it will offer more options than "male" and "female") and marriage (while it can be important for legal and insurance reasons to know whether a patient is legally married, many members of sexual minorities are part of non-traditional relationships – multipartner arrangements, same-sex marriages, owner/slave agreements – and the health care practitioner should be aware of these as well).

Physicians have a reputation for being politically conservative, and it's probably true that there are more Republican doctors than Democratic ones. Even in San Francisco, I have encountered quite a few doctors who are somewhere to the right of Genghis Khan. What has been truly amazing to me is that while these doctors might personally disapprove of what you do, they will still give you excellent medical care. I still refer patients to these physicians – I don't care about their politics and they don't care about mine (except once in a while in the physicians' dining room, but that's another story).

How do you find a practitioner? If you don't currently have a physician with whom you feel comfortable, you may have to look around to find one.

Today, many people belong to HMOs (health maintenance organizations), which we discussed in the last chapter. In these systems, physicians are paid a set fee for each patient every month, whether they see that patient or not. Obviously, the physician with healthy patients will make money, and the one with patients who need frequent visits will lose money. Doctors, like most of us, do not want to work harder than necessary. Thus, a patient who looks as though she'll be demanding or hard to work with may find it hard to find a welcoming physician. HMO rules try to prevent doctors from refusing patients who are sick, but there are ways around these rules. Doctors may assume that a patient who is a member of a sexual minority is likely to be difficult. (You may say you wouldn't want a physician like that – but you probably also don't want a physician who is too busy to give you the time you need.) If the physician has to invest a lot of time learning about your sexual lifestyle, whether or not you are a "difficult" patient, the physician may choose to be less than welcoming.

It is thus in your best interests, when choosing a physician, to present yourself as sane, self-aware and sensible. The following suggestions are not meant to teach you how to be a good patient, nor do they imply that sexual minorities are bad patients. Many sexual minorities have avoided traditional health care for so long that they do not know how the system works these days.

A good way to start is to ask others in your sexual community for recommendations. If other practitioners of your sexual behavior and/or lifestyle are happy with their medical care, then it's a pretty good bet that you will be, too. In addition, such referrals tend to reward nonjudgmental physicians by sending them lots of new patients.

Some people split their care so that they go to a nearby physician for non-sexual issues, but travel some distance to a sex-positive physician for their sexual matters. This may be the best approach if you can't find a nonjudgmental doctor in your area, or if you do not trust the confidentiality of local doctors.

However, if your health insurance requires you to pick one doctor, then you have to make some choices. If you choose the nearby doctor as your primary care physician, you'll probably wind up having to pay the sex-positive doctor out of pocket. On the other hand, if you designate the sex-positive doctor as your primary care physician, then you wind up making a long, uncomfortable drive for minor flus, headaches and infections – and a "short" forty-minute drive can seem very long indeed when you're fighting an intestinal virus.

What if you go to a clinic? If you get your health care from a clinic, you may not always have the same physician, or you may have a limited choice of physicians. Get to know the administrator/nurses/receptionists at the clinic, and see if they can clue you into which doctors are likely to be accepting. You do not have to describe your behavior or lifestyle, but it is more likely that someone open about sex generally would be open about your kink, whatever it is.

Finding out about the practitioner you already have. If you already have a health care practitioner with whom you are basically comfortable, but you're not sure whether or not he is nonjudgmental about sexuality and alternative sexual behaviors, make an appointment for a consultation. Pay for this appointment as you would any other; because you are paying, you get to ask your questions. You can start off with a statement like "I have not told you about all the sexual activities in which I engage. I want to be honest with you, and I have some medical questions about how these activities can impact my health." If you notice your doctor squirming, or a change in the way she interacts with you, it is time to consider changing doctors.

If the direct approach is too confrontational for you, you can start by asking third party questions: "I have a friend who is involved in kinky sex and needs a doctor. How open are you about inviting such people into your practice?"

If you are seeking a new physician, an interview is appropriate. Most ethical health care practitioners should be willing to give you five minutes for a short interview. I do not charge for this consultation, but other physicians feel that a token payment is important. Do be sensitive to the reality that most health care practitioners must care for dozens of patients a day and are chronically rushed – please keep it brief, accept a telephone interview if it's offered, and realize that the appointment may need to be at the convenience of the practitioner.

Do *not* try to get medical advice during this interview; that's not its purpose. It's OK to ask if the doctor has had much experience treating HIV or lupus or what-have-you (or what-you-have), but asking "what do you think these red bumps are?" during an informational interview is stealing medical advice. In addition, a physician who diagnoses without a history and careful examination is not someone you want taking care of you.

Here are four "litmus test" questions you can ask. You'll be able to tell quite a bit from the answers you get, as well as from the practitioner's demeanor as she answers you.

1.   *"How do you feel about non-monogamous sexual relationships?"* You yourself don't have to be interested in non-monogamy to ask this question; it's simply a way to find out how open your practitioner is to non-traditional sexualities. An answer that might signal sex-negativity would be one that uses words like "promiscuous" or "adultery," or that otherwise implies that non-monogamous relationships are inherently sinful or damaging. A better answer might be one that focuses on the consent of everybody involved, and/or on disease prevention strategies.

2.   *"How do you personally feel about masturbation?"* Uptight or sex-negative practitioners will give, predictably, uptight or sex-negative answers to this question. They may focus on sex addiction or intimacy-avoidance issues, or simply seem uncomfortable with the whole idea. The sex-positive practitioner knows that masturbation is a normal, healthy sexual outlet engaged in by most people, as well as an excellent safer-sex strategy, and will tell you so. She may reject masturbation personally, but the question is how she does it – there's a big difference between "I'm Catholic so it's not acceptable for me" and "It's a sin against God." It's also quite reasonable for her to answer "I prefer not to talk about my personal beliefs," but follow up with, "What do you think about your patients who do?" Negativity in this answer is not acceptable.

3.   *"I'm into some unusual sexual behaviors. How do you feel about that?"* If you get an offhanded reply of "Oh, that's fine with me," you may have a problem. Not all unusual sexual behaviors are OK, from either a legal or a medical standpoint; if you're into something that could seriously damage your health, your health care practitioner needs to know that. A better answer might be, "What kind of sexual behaviors?" A comment like, "Do not tell me about illegal sexual behaviors or behaviors that I am required to report to the authorities, such as sex with children, unless you want to be reported," is reasonable and honest.

One acquaintance of mine, a therapist who specializes in handling bizarre sexual cases, was talking to a patient whose fetish was handling raw meat: "I feel all the packages of meat until I find the one I like best, then take it home, fuck it, cook it and eat it for dinner." He then named his favorite butcher counter, which happened to be the same one frequented by the therapist. It's circumstances like these which prove that even the most liberal of us will encounter challenges to our open-mindedness.

4.   *"What would you do if you found marks on my body?"* If the practitioner replies "Nothing," or "That'd be fine with me," you might want to investigate further. A better answer might be, "I'd ask how you got them." It's part of your health care practitioner's job to make sure you're not being abused or harmed, and unless you explain, he has no way of knowing whether those bruises were consensually given by a loving partner,

or the aftermath of a rape or assault. On the other hand, if the physician is upset at the thought of finding marks on your body at all, she might not be your best choice as a doctor.

If you feel comfortable with your practitioner's answers to these four questions, and if she is a good fit for you in terms of her specialty, her reputation, and her ability to work with your finances (insurance, HMOs, governmental support, or private payment), you may have found yourself a health care practitioner.

What if you can't find a sex-positive practitioner? Let's suppose that after a reasonable search you cannot find a physician who is a good fit for you. All is not lost.

First, let's hope that this is an unusual situation. Smoking is a much more medically damaging behavior than most sexual activities. Most physicians are aware of the medical problems with smoking, are not happy to have smokers in their practice (they have more visits and use more resources, a no-no under managed care) – but smokers still do find good, competent medical care.

Second, it's worth taking a second look at your criteria. Did you pass up someone who wasn't perfect but who would and could give you reasonable care?

If you're still stuck, there are other avenues to explore. Try asking your insurance company. You don't have to give the details – "I'm a female-to-male transsexual trying to get pregnant and nobody will help me." You could say, "I have a unique appearance and I am looking for a physician who will not prejudge me on that appearance." Insurance companies want to make you happy and tend to know who is in their network. They may be able to refer you to someone.

Or go to the hospital you wish to use and ask to see a nurse. Do *not* sign in, and be understanding if they are too busy at that time – come back at another time. The nurse can be a supervisor, in the urgent care clinic, or even in the emergency room. The nurses tend to know the physicians with whom they work, so they might be able to suggest someone to you.

You can try being open with a physician you suspect may be judgmental. Inform her before the appointment that you are there to ask some questions and do not want this appointment recorded in your chart. If you are a confident and competent practitioner of an alternative sexual lifestyle, you will challenge many of the physician's stereotypes; she may come to think of you as the exception that proves the rule, but you will get good care. If you find that she is so judgmental that she cannot offer you good care, it might be safest to pay her out of pocket rather than taking a chance that negative information about you could go into your permanent insurance files.

However, this choice is not always as easy as it sounds. Many sexual advocacy groups suggest "coming out" as a mechanism for fostering acceptance. If this idea fits your political perspective, it may be worth trying. If you are wrong, you can always change physicians. (We'll talk about *how* to come out to your physician in the next chapter.)

If you're still stuck, you may have to accept the idea of working with a physician with whom you cannot be *completely* open. Search for a sex-positive physician in a more distant location, and use him for your sexual issues. With your local doctor, it is perfectly acceptable to refuse to discuss the details of your sex life, although it's clearly not the best possible solution. (You might consider lending or anonymously sending her a copy of this book.) However, in some specific situations, you may need to respond to direct questions that are medically relevant. It is permissible to ask why that piece of information is important.

Do not give up the search. You deserve, and it is your right to have, competent, nonjudgmental medical care. As medicine grapples with sexual issues, physicians will change, even in the most conservative parts of the country. Remember, even during the years when African-Americans in the South were hideously oppressed, there were white physicians who cared for them, even when it cost them their white patients. Sexual minorities are no different, and no less deserving.

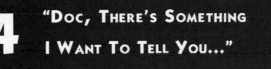

4 "Doc, There's Something I Want To Tell You…"

John and Tara had been playing together in a committed consensual owner/slave relationship for several months. Although both were married to others, their respective spouses were happy that they had found such an appropriate outlet for John's dominant desires and Tara's deep submissiveness. John and Tara were committed to one another in an intimate way – possibly with even greater intimacy than to their legal spouses.

This couple was first "referred" to me from the Internet. John had sent out an SOS to an S/M-oriented mailing list and someone suggested he e-mail me. After their last play date, which included some mutually pleasurable caning of her breasts, Tara had developed some worrisome symptoms: one breast was swollen, hot, red and hard to the touch. She hadn't been to a doctor in years – she was afraid that her lifestyle, and the subsequent marks on her body, would create problems. She feared the moralizing tone and disapproval that she felt were inevitable. It was easier to ignore the whole thing.

Needless to say, I sent back an immediate e-mail strongly advising that they see a physician quickly. They lived on another coast and could not see me. After some cajoling, she went to a medical doctor. A mammogram and subsequent biopsy revealed a cancer in the affected breast.

John and Tara found themselves plunged into a nightmare. She had no physician to advocate for her interests. The specialists did not understand or respect the relationship between John and Tara, and wanted to deal only with Tara's legal husband. John felt miserably guilty: he thought that he had caused Tara's cancer by his caning of her breasts over the months of their relationship – despite my assurance that the cancer had taken root long before he and Tara had begun playing. He also felt cut off from Tara, excluded by her physicians from the frank discussions and treatment decisions. Most of this would not have happened if Tara had established a relationship with a nonjudgmental primary care physician before she started having problems.

How to do it. Coming out – forthrightly sharing information about your sexual orientation and/or practices – to your doctor, chiropractor, physician's assistant, nurse practitioner or other health-care provider probably won't be quite as tough as coming out to your mother. But it won't be easy either.

While I (obviously) think of myself as a sex-positive physician, there are patients I've taken care of for many years who were not able to confide that they were gay, or even that they enjoyed oral sex. Others cannot tell me they are having concerns about their sexual functioning, even when they're feeling quite distressed about it.

Doctors often talk about the "hand-on-the-doorknob question." As the practitioner finishes with the original purpose of the appointment and is getting ready to leave the room, just as his hand reaches the doorknob, the patient says, "Oh, doctor, just one more question…." And then the *real* issue emerges. Due to the sensitivity of these issues and/or the patient's shyness about making explicit statements, this question often takes up much more time than the original appointment, as the practitioner must take the appropriate history and fully explain the patient's options. Given that most patients in today's health care system are only allotted fifteen minutes or less for an appointment, dealing with sexual concerns can put a real "kink" (not the good kind) in a practitioner's schedule. It works better for you and for your health care practitioner if you can schedule a special appointment to discuss your sexual concerns. You'll probably find that you will get better information and more attention if you ask your real question right after the doctor comes into the room instead of as she's about to leave it. Many of my patients find it useful to make a list of their concerns before they come in to see me, so they can be sure that their nervousness will not cause them to overlook anything important.

As a physician, I'm often tempted to help a patient come out. They usually start off with "I have something to tell you," then begin to stammer and, very slowly and obliquely, come to the point. (My experience is that the more conventional the behavior they're trying to tell me about, the harder a time they have talking about it: one young woman took two entire appointments trying to tell me that she thought she was a lesbian.) I can certainly sympathize with how difficult it can be to come out to a relative stranger; it can be hard not to save them this discomfort by asking them a direct question. Yet any time I do, I wind up stepping in it.

I remember a man – long-haired, with manicured nails, and dressed in a pink ruffled shirt – who said that he was uncomfortable with the demands of the male role. Over the next ten minutes, he told me that he wanted to radically change his life and sexuality. Yet when I gently suggested that he might be transgendered, he was very surprised and offended and wanted to know how I'd gotten that idea: he was *trying* to tell me that he was having problems getting erections.

I share this story to remind us all that we cannot divine each other's thoughts: even if your health care provider is very knowledgeable about alternative sexualities, it's up to you to be forthright about the information you're trying to share.

I practice in San Francisco, a city well known for its acceptance of non-traditional sexual behavior and lifestyles. Many people tell me that they are completely "out" concerning their sexual behavior: if their physician can't handle it, it's the doctor's problem, not theirs. While that is one perspective, I think it's a much better idea to have patient and physician working together. Additionally, a nonjudgmental physician is more likely to be able to give you helpful information to help make whatever activity or lifestyle you choose safer and more satisfactory.

You may be afraid that the practitioner will judge you or lecture you or just give you a funny look. Or you may be afraid of worse: that he will report you to the police, or your insurance company, or your employer, or your family. Most health care practitioners take their confidentiality obligations very seriously, and will not share any information unnecessarily. Your job is to help make sure that nobody feels it necessary to share that information – and you can help do that by coming out to your physician carefully, sanely and with accurate information.

Imagine the difference, for the average physician, between:

"My lover and I are into cock & ball torture, and I don't want to deny him anything. I couldn't stand it if he left me or found someone else, but I'm afraid that he'll do something so extreme that it will injure me permanently."

And: "I love it when my lover very roughly stimulates my genitals. Nevertheless, I am concerned about the long-term effects of this behavior."

How to talk about sex. For almost everybody, talking about sex is hard, difficult, uncomfortable, unpleasant, upsetting, and not the way you really want to spend your time.

I've been a sex educator for decades and a doctor for quite a few years, and even I often find it difficult to talk about sex – not because I am embarrassed, but because the words often do not exist with which to ask nonjudgmental questions. Sometimes people are offended when I ask if they take part in some particular behavior, others are offended if the questions do not use the correct jargon ("How dare you call me submissive? I am the wholly owned slave of my master!" "I am not a lesbian, I have never even been to the Greek island of Lesbos – I am a butch dyke and don't you forget it.") Similarly, my non-sexual-minority patients can be offended when I ask about alternative sexuality.

Please recognize that nobody can guess someone's private sexual behavior from their outside appearance or even by their stated sexual orientation; if your doctor doesn't ask, she will probably make incorrect assumptions. Please be as open as you can: "Doctor, I know I am 85 years old, but I am concerned that the cause of my sore throat might be a sexually transmitted disease. Can you make sure the antibiotic you are prescribing will cover that?"

Many people joke about sex easily, but when it is time to be serious, most fall quiet. Our culture teaches us that it's not appropriate to be straightforward – outside the bedroom, or even inside it – when discussing our sexual desires and behaviors. It is often a major accomplishment to be able to tell your partner what you desire sexually.

Keeping frank sexual talk in the bedroom is fine, if that's what you want... with one exception: your doctor's office. You *must* tell your health care practitioner about any sexual behaviors that might be affecting your health. He cannot provide you with an acceptable level of care if he doesn't have enough information to do so. Several people have paid for an hour of my time just to ask me questions about the medical ramifications of their specific sexual practices and to garner suggestions about how to do them more safely.

If you find it hard to say the words, write a few notes to yourself before you go in, so you don't forget important information in the embarrassment of the moment. Some patients give me a letter to read in their presence, send me an e-mail, or just blush their way through a face-to-face conversation.

Just because you have an accepting physician does not mean you necessarily have to come out immediately with every detail of your sexual behavior. It is quite appropriate to start by simply giving your doctor enough information to begin discussing the health risks, if any, of your activities. Later, as the doctor/patient relationship strengthens, then you may feel more comfortable sharing more details.

When to come out. You will get better care if you come out to your physician during a regular appointment. If you wait until you're in some kind of crisis (a stuck butt plug, a bleeding laceration, a badly infected piercing, whatever), you are putting your doctor into a difficult position. For one thing, there's no guarantee that your doctor will be the one on call when the fecal matter hits the ventilation device, and the physician who is on call may or may not be open-minded – the result will be your physician hearing the events from his uptight associate.

Also, it's only fair to give your health care practitioner a chance to learn more about your sexual practices – and to voice objections, if he has any – before a serious problem arises. A calm discussion when no problem exists is more likely to be successful than confronting your physician with an injury or illness resulting from your sexual behavior – a busy and worried doctor is less likely to be sympathetic to discussions of "safe, sane and consensual."

A better time to come out is either during the initial interview we discussed last chapter, or during your first appointment. During this discussion, it's very important that you keep in mind what your statements may sound like to someone who doesn't live in the same community you do. I spoke to one woman on the Internet who was terribly upset because a new doctor had expressed concern that she might be mentally ill and/or an abuse victim. "He asked about the piercings in my nipples," she related. "I told him that my master had put them there for his own pleasure." She had apparently gone on to explain that she had no say in the procedure, and that she was wholly devoted to pleasing her master by accepting any pain or marks he desired. To this woman, the piercings were a lovely romantic symbol of her devotion – but to the physician, they (understandably) sounded like abuse. Yet if she'd simply said, "I like the way they look, and so does my partner," the piercings would probably have gotten no additional notice at all.

This would also have given the woman a good opening to start talking to her doctor about her relationship and behaviors. Here's the conversation I *wish* had taken place:

Doctor: I notice that you have jewelry in your nipples. Can I ask what led you to having them pierced?

Patient: Yes. I like the way they look, and so does my partner.

Doctor: Are you having any problems with infection or discharge?

Patient: No. It went so well that I'm also thinking about additional piercings.

Doctor: May I ask where?

Patient: Sure, but first I'd like to discuss some other aspects of my sexual history. My partner and I are involved in an S/M relationship. Do you know what that is?

Doctor: Not really.

Patient: We role-play a variety of scenes during sex. Sometimes, as a result, I have bruises and other marks on my body. I wanted to tell you this before you actually saw it and became concerned that I was being abused. What we do is consensual, and I have never enjoyed sex or a relationship so much.

Doctor: To be honest, I don't really know very much about this sort of thing.

Patient: I can refer you to some reading materials if you're interested. And to answer your other question, I want my clitoral hood pierced.

Doctor: I don't know anything about that or its possible complications.

Patient: If it becomes infected or causes any other problems, I will come in immediately.

Doctor: OK.

It is part of the physician's job to understand that abuse and violence happen, and to protect his patients from being abused. Abuse is not the exclusive province of vanilla heterosexuals; gays, lesbians, transgendered folk, polyamorists, sex workers and S/M people can also be the victims of abuse – so if your health care provider asks questions that sound like she's wondering whether or not you're being abused, that doesn't mean she's a clueless prude, it means she's doing her best to take care of you.

Does your doctor really need to know all about your slave contract or your cocksucking technique or your rubber fetish? Not unless they affect your health. A good patient has at least some boundaries regarding what information is appropriate to share with her physician: a great way to alienate your doctor is to tell him just before your pelvic exam that your number-one fantasy is to be subjected to painful medical procedures by a sadistic physician. (Yes, it's happened to me.)

On the other hand, it's extremely important to be honest with your health care practitioner. If she asks you whether you engage in oral-anal contact (rimming), that's not because she's getting off on the thought – it's because rimming has specific medical meanings in terms of its effect on your health, and she needs to know the answer to her question so she can appropriately order specific tests. Lying or evasiveness frustrates your doctor and can harm your health.

Start by saying, "There's some information you need to have about me." Then, simply describe any alternative sexual behaviors that could have any effect on your health or well-being. You should touch on:

-      What kind(s) of sex you typically have (vaginal, anal, oral, fisting, etc.)

- Your safer sex precautions and techniques

- The number of partners with whom you have sexual contact and other erotic activities

- Any activities that might involve bruising or breaking the skin

- Any activities that are potentially risky to your health (breath control, electricity, fireplay, ingestion of feces, etc.)

- Any body modifications

- Drug or alcohol use patterns

- Birth control methods (including "none")

- Any unusual family structures or relationships (polyamorous, owner/slave, etc.) which should be taken into account for hospital visitation, decision-making and so on

- Anybody in your family structure who doesn't know about these activities and should be shielded from this information

Be sure to update this information periodically.

Throughout this discussion, emphasize that you choose these behaviors of your own free will, that you do them for your personal enjoyment, and that you have taken the time to educate yourself about how to do them as safely as possible. Try to be sensitive to your physician's body language, and not give too much information all at once: if this is to be an ongoing relationship, you don't want her first impression to be "that man who made me feel really uncomfortable" or worse. This first "coming-out" appointment may not be the best time to discuss the specific safety measures that you use, but you should probably find a time to talk about them during subsequent appointments.

Your health care practitioner should be asking straightforward questions which can be answered simply. If she wants more information about *why* you do such things, a simple "because I enjoy it" should suffice; there are no real answers to "why" questions. She does not need to know the heartfelt details of your love for your three spouses or the specific color and design of your favorite high heels; she just needs to know what you're doing that could have ramifications to your health.

What if she insists on prying into irrelevant stuff, or expresses harsh judgments about your behavior? This is a good time for an assertive attitude: "That sounded very judgmental; are you upset about what I do?" Your health care practitioner is there to help you; she doesn't get to make you feel uncomfortable.

Nonetheless, physicians in general are curious people, and when confronted with something they have never seen before are likely to ask questions. Some of these questions may be clueless, just like the ones you've been asked elsewhere in the straight world. If you feel like answering them, go ahead – but be sure to make it clear that you're speaking for yourself only and not for anyone else who shares your sexual kinks; it's not a good idea to let your doctor generalize what she's learned about you to all the other sexual minority members in the world. Rather than spending your own and your physician's time teaching Alternative Sexualities 101 from the exam table, consider suggesting that she obtain and read a couple of the excellent books on the topic; several are listed in the Resource Guide.

Some people engage in behaviors that are technically or actually illegal in their locale (such as sodomy or prostitution), or jobs with questionable societal acceptance (such as stripper, lingerie model, professional dominatrix). While such individuals may be concerned about having this kind of information on an official record, your physician can't help you if he doesn't know. If you state your concern in the beginning, your physician *may* be able to record your medical issues and concerns without specifically stating your involvement in the worrisome (to you) behavior.

Similarly, drug users may be concerned (with some cause) about anyone recording their admission in an official document. Some drug users may also find that their doctors are reluctant to prescribe certain psychoactive drugs, such as narcotics, for fear that the patient will abuse the medication. You can and should discuss your concern with your doctor without telling her the specifics. Physicians will, almost universally, tell you what they feel compelled to record and what they will discuss "off the record." That discussion may well lead to a frank talk about your sexual behavior and what problems can occur when you use substances while engaging in sex.

What are the risks? Some people are hesitant to come out to their health care practitioners because they're afraid they'll be "outed" to their families, employers, insurance companies, or even the police.

In most cases, these fears are groundless. Health care practitioners are very careful and serious about matters of confidentiality; we take our patients' trust seriously. However, you should be aware of some exceptions.

If you are describing behavior that involves sex with, or abuse of, a minor, your health care practitioner must by law report you to the proper authorities. The same rules apply if you are engaging in abuse of a dependent adult (someone who is mentally retarded, or frail and elderly), or if you threaten to do harm to yourself or someone else. Please be assured that you *will* be reported if you describe any of these behaviors.

If, in your health care practitioner's opinion, your activities represent an immediate danger to yourself or others, he can have you involuntarily committed to a mental institution for observation and evaluation. This is very rare.

Health care practitioners are also required to report certain infections, including sexually transmitted diseases, to the Health Department. The purpose of this reporting is to prevent the spread of these diseases, not to out you to anyone; the people who work for health departments also take your privacy very seriously. If they disclosed confidential information they would have even more difficulty getting cooperation from the people they were interviewing, thus defeating their purpose.

With these few exceptions, we are not required to report anything else. I have never heard of a patient being reported to the police by a health care practitioner for consensual behavior with another non-dependent adult.

When you sign up with an insurance company, you sign a release that gives the insurers access to your records. There is nothing the health care practitioner can do to prevent this access. (In my office, HIV records are kept in separate files, but we can't have double files on every disease or for individual situations.) The insurance company probably doesn't give a damn whether or not you like to be spanked, and they *do* have a responsibility to keep this information private. If you are still concerned about confidentiality, the way to take maximum precautions is to see the health care practitioner under an assumed name, and pay cash. If you do that, there's no way your insurance company or your employer can get hold of your private information. Unfortunately, that is a very expensive alternative.

As for your family, they have no legal right to your medical information. If you've been straight (pardon the expression) with your doctor about who knows what, he can help keep information from those who shouldn't have it, and he may be able to help get it to those who should – including those who might not be part of your traditional family structure. If you are involved in a nontraditional relationship or family, please execute a power of attorney for health care and a living will. A general durable power of attorney and a will are also excellent ideas. Actually, even if you are in a traditional relationship, you should make your desires known and execute these documents.

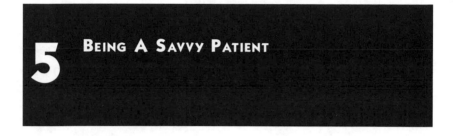

5 BEING A SAVVY PATIENT

Back in Chapter Two, I explained some of the basics of today's health care environment. My personal opinions about managed care and its ramifications, or about the state of government-supported health care programs, aren't too relevant here; neither, sadly, are yours. The fact is that for many if not most people these days, these programs are a reality – which means that getting the best care from your physician or other health care provider means knowing a bit about how the system works and about how you can work well within the system.

In recent years, the cost of running a medical practice has increased and the reimbursement the physician receives has decreased. While few physicians are on the welfare lines, we are having to look more carefully than ever before at our bottom line – and many of us are getting very frustrated (early retirement among physicians is increasing exponentially). Thus, one of the important criteria physicians use in deciding which patients are desirable is how efficiently those patients use their services.

But that's certainly not the only goal. Physicians like to cure things; it's why we're physicians. So if you are really sick, but the physician can save your life, end your pain once and for all, fix something so it never bothers you again, or manage a chronic illness so that it has as little impact on your life as possible, you will be a favored patient. You are a walking billboard to your physician's skill (even if she is the only one to recognize it). Thus, the cooperative patient who complies with the physician's recommendations and is open to various alternatives is likely to have a happy and hard-working physician.

Mr. Jones, a forty-three-year-old obese white male, smokes two packs of cigarettes a day, says he rarely drinks but on further questioning admits has five drinks every Friday or Saturday, has sky-high cholesterol and a father who died of a heart attack at age forty-five. He rarely exercises and his blood pressure is moderately elevated, but he is not diabetic (at least not yet). Modern medicine can greatly decrease his risk of heart attack and stroke: the treatment involves medication *and* lifestyle changes. Mr. Jones insists on trying diet changes first, before any medication or other lifestyle changes, in spite of having failed at numerous diets in the past. He has now become either a project or a lost cause – most likely the latter. Mr. Jones is a managed care "success": he's using no medication and few resources. Patients change insurance plans so often that he will probably have his heart attack on another plan. However, his disease process continues unabated and his doctor – who went to medical school to learn to help people get healthier – gets increasingly cynical and/or frustrated.

There is a reason why this explanation is included in a book like this. Individuals may assume that the reason they have not found an "understanding" physician is due to her moral concerns related to their sexual behavior. While this is undoubtedly the case for some physicians, other considerations may also play a significant role. The premise of this book is that everyone is entitled to nonjudgmental health care, so below are some suggestions on how to get the most out of your health care provider and to ensure a mutually satisfying relationship.

1.   *Know why you are going to the doctor.* Even the most liberal and open-minded physician can only do what he is trained to do. Asking your traditionally trained physician about herbal remedies is likely to get a clueless answer: very little research has been done on herbs, so even the most accepting physician can only say things like "this herb has helped a lot of my patients" or "many other practitioners find this herb helpful in situations like yours." (Some physicians do work closely with naturopaths and other herbal healers and can refer you to them for help.) If you want herbal advice, your mainstream physician is unlikely to have the answer. On the other hand, all medications, including herbal remedies, have side effects: don't assume the side effects you are experiencing are from the prescription medication you are taking rather than the herbs. You must tell your physician about any herbal remedies you are using, since this information is relevant in diagnosing your problem and prescribing other medications.

2.   *Know your health history.* Before you go to a new physician, be sure you know the names and dosages of any medications you might be taking (handing your doctor a written list is great), any allergies you might have to medications, food or environmental factors, and the name and address of your previous caregiver.

3.   *Be careful with your laundry list of problems.* If you go to the physician, perhaps for the first time in a long time, with a list of twenty problems to be addressed, none of them can be addressed completely. Focus on one problem at a time. Recognize that it may take a few appointments to get to the bottom of your list: if you go to a contractor with twelve things that need to be fixed on your house, she may feel that it's more important to fix the leaky roof right away than to cover up that terrible pink paint in your living room, even if the pink paint is driving you nuts. The problem that bothers you most may not be the problem that your doctor focuses on: "I know you are very upset about the appearance of your toenails, especially since your partner gets off on sucking your toes – but the shortness of breath, sweating, chest pressure, and numbness down your left arm every time you take a brisk walk is more important to address right now." The patient who has dangerously high blood pressure, and who never calls for refills on his blood pressure medication but never misses a refill on his skin cream, is a disaster waiting to happen.

4.   *Respect your doctor's limits.* A former patient of mine moved across the country and had to find a new physi-

cian. She found one who seemed open, so she asked him, "Do you have any problem with the fact that I practice consensual dominance and submission?" He quickly responded "No," then thought a minute and added, "As long as you aren't into that asphyxiation stuff." Arguing at that point about why choking scenes turned her on was not likely to have much effect. Instead, a simple "Well, I do enjoy that, so I will seek another physician," was a more reasonable response. This doctor did a good job of stating his limits, and the patient did a good job of respecting them. (Just for the record, asphyxiation scenes are more dangerous than many people realize – so if you insist on doing them, recognize that you may be sustaining cumulative damage.)

5. *Understand the time constraints.* As stated earlier, the only way to make a living in managed care is to increase one's panel of patients. By doing so, the physician takes on the responsibility of taking care of those patients. As the number of patients increase, so does the pressure to decrease the time spent with each patient. Most physicians try to see four to six patients per hour, and some try to see more – so, at best, you have fifteen minutes with the physician. You can help speed the appointment along by being organized, knowing what information you want to give your doctor, perhaps even making a few notes ahead of time so that you can tell him what he needs to know as quickly as possible.

Obviously, if you are sick, the physician will spend as much time as necessary with you, but routine appointments can seem rushed. While it can be infuriating to have to come back for routine issues (and pay another copayment – physicians are not allowed to waive this fee), it is the system: your doctor almost certainly hates it as much as you do, maybe even more.

Also, please try to be understanding if your doctor is running a little late for your appointment. While most doctors do their best to maintain a timely schedule, genuine emergencies can and do happen and can wreak havoc on a physician's promptness. Your doctor's office may try to contact you if they know your appointment will be delayed, but they may not be able to reach you in time.

6. *Don't ask the physician to bend the HMO rules for you.* You (and/or your employer) picked your insurance plan. It may be bare bones and not cover very much, but there isn't much your doctor can do about that. Bending the rules for you – for example, fudging on the name of the procedure she's performed so that it can be covered by your insurance – puts her in a very awkward position. Physicians literally run out of hours in the day fighting for medically essential procedures for their sickest patients; insisting that they take that time obtaining authorization for a procedure not covered by your plan is not ethical or honest. You and your doctor are both working within a not-very-hospitable system; please help her out by understanding her position.

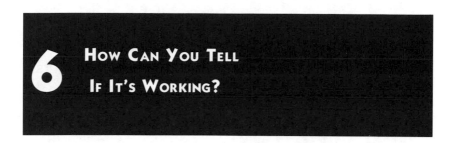

6 HOW CAN YOU TELL
IF IT'S WORKING?

A good relationship between a patient and a health care practitioner should offer a reasonably high level of comfort, communication and trust for everybody involved. Here are some checkpoints to use to see whether your health care relationship is working well – from *both* points of view.

From the patient's point of view:

You feel comfortable, or at least able to begin, discussing intimate sexual matters with your health care practitioner. You feel equally open about discussing other potentially controversial areas of your life, such as drug use, alternative lifestyle choices and so on.

Overall, you feel that your health care practitioner accepts your sexual practices as an informed choice. She is able to explain the medical ramifications of your choices without making negative judgments about them beyond that. A good rule of thumb is that you should feel you can tell your physician about a planned sexual behavior, with the expectation that she will explain the possible health repercussions of the behavior.

You don't withhold information because you're afraid of what your health care practitioner might say.

You don't have a knot in your stomach when you think about going to the health care practitioner. (Of course, some people are always nervous about a trip to the doctor – but nervousness beyond what you usually feel may be a sign of trouble.)

You feel that you can be yourself around your health care practitioner. You don't feel that you should put on a special outfit, different from your everyday clothes, to visit your health care practitioner. (Wearing clothes that are relatively easy to remove and put back on is a courteous touch. And going out of your way to be shocking or seductive toward your doctor, or toward his staff or patients in the waiting room, is inappropriate.)

Your health care practitioner is aware of your family and relationship structures, and is aware of any relevant legal documentations such as living wills or durable powers of attorney for health care.

The office staff is courteous, friendly and helpful to you – even if they can't always give you the 2:45 appointment that fits into your hectic schedule.

Your health care practitioner usually returns calls the same day you place them, and fills prescriptions in a timely manner (within two days). You can help by making sure that your prescriptions don't run out over a weekend.

Your health care practitioner listens to you and doesn't discount your symptoms or opinions, whether or not she agrees with you.

Your health care practitioner treats you as part of your own health care team.

You trust your health care practitioner.

From your health care practitioner's point of view:

You are honest about your sexual behaviors and practices and have a sense of what information is important to share.

You answer questions straightforwardly and readily.

You recognize that your practitioner can't read your mind – if she isn't going to make assumptions about you (assuming, for example, that a woman wearing a "Dyke Power" button doesn't have sex with men), she may have to ask you some questions. You don't take offense at those questions.

You are friendly and courteous with the office staff and with other patients you may encounter in the health care practitioner's office. You don't behave or dress seductively or outrageously toward them. You don't expect the office staff to drop everything to deal with your problems.

You are organized in giving information to your doctor. You communicate your health care issues efficiently, not waiting until the appointment is almost over to mention something important.

If your health care practitioner does something or expresses herself in some way that you don't like, you speak up promptly, clearly and politely so that she has a chance to rectify the error, or to explain the reason she behaved the way she did. (Even the best health care practitioner does not "click" with every patient. The problem might be hers, yours, or a simple mismatch of personalities. If you don't click, that's not the same thing as the physician being incompetent or clueless; find other help if you need to, but bad-mouthing the physician without good reason is inappropriate.)

If your health care practitioner does something or expresses himself in some way that you *do* like, you thank him!

You don't judge your health care practitioner on the basis of his gender, age, orientation, race or background.

You have appropriate personal boundaries regarding your relationship with your health care practitioner.

If you are aware of your health care practitioner's own sexual orientation or practices, you respect his confidentiality when speaking to his colleagues, staff and other patients.

You are careful about your hygiene, keeping your body as clean as possible when you come to your health care practitioner's office. Avoiding artificial scents, which may cause problems for other patients, is thoughtful.

If you can answer most of the questions on both of these checklists with a "Yes," then you're doing great. Congratulations!

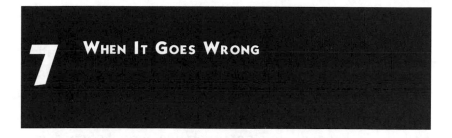

7 WHEN IT GOES WRONG

Most relationships between a health care practitioner and a patient are respectful, professional, and well-bounded. But doctor-patient relationships can be challenging.

Your physician is close to you in ways that other people aren't – she examines your body closely, touches areas no one else touches, causes pain and discomfort, explores areas of your body and psyche that nobody else can. And people with alternative sexualities are often concerned – occasionally with cause – that their sexuality may make them vulnerable to improper treatment by an unscrupulous physician.

On the other hand, some patients exhibit remarkably bad boundaries with their physicians. One of my S/M-identified female patients responded to every question with a "yes sir" or "no sir" until I firmly told her to stop, and another actually requested that I masturbate her during her pelvic exam. And then there are the patients who show up in my waiting room crossdressed in a see-through shirt and nipple rings, and happily assure the elderly couple waiting to see my colleague that "Everybody *loves* Dr. Moser." The only way for an ethical health care practitioner to respond to such behavior is with a polite but firm insistence that it stop.

Physicians today are the targets of many lawsuits, some over mistaken sexual intentions. Perhaps the best way to alienate your physician is to place him or her in a situation where sexual intent can be ambiguous. Most physicians have had passes made at them, and most know how to politely decline. Nonetheless, it is not always clear how to respond, and medical school does not teach this aspect of care very well.

If you feel any sense of sexual unease with your health care practitioner, it's time for a frank discussion. Whether or not your discomfort has a factual basis, letting him know that you're feeling uncomfortable can help guide him toward taking care of you in a way that feels better to you.

I often have female patients who request to be nude, dispensing with sheets and gowns, during their exam; they feel that this choice humanizes the exam, makes it less clinical and enabling the practitioner to treat the patient holistically. For many, this is a comfortable and empowering experience. Others, unfortunately, feel intimidated by a fully dressed man examining a naked female, and may feel ashamed of what they see as a "political" failure; when I sense their ambivalence and offer them a cover, they refuse and go on feeling unhappy. An uncomfortable patient makes for an uncomfortable physician, which can lead to misunderstandings. A few physicians find a nude patient to be beyond their own personal limits, and should have these limits respected.

Once, when examining a new female patient, I noticed a large fleshy mole on her breast, right where it could be irritated by her bra. I innocently asked, pointing to the mole, "Does this bother you?" She replied, "No, I'm quite comfortable being examined by male physicians." I was, of course, able to explain the intent of my question, but the exchange did remind me that anything a doctor says or does can be misunderstood.

Some people choose a physician because they have sexual issues with the examination. I have lesbian patients who choose me because an exam by another woman would feel too sexual to them. Others feel comfortable with me for all exams except pelvics. Do what feels comfortable to you – your health care should make you feel better, not worse. Of course, there are times when your discomfort is less important than your continuing good health: sometimes a pelvic exam, rectal exam or other procedure is necessary to deal with an urgent problem. However, in the absence of a very good reason why, nobody should make you feel uncomfortable – even if your discomfort isn't related to any purposeful action by your practitioner.

By the way, back in Chapter One I talked about the schizophrenic quality of my medical school training regarding pelvic exams – which, of course, brings up the question of how a physician *can* do a pelvic exam in an appropriately professional and non-sexual manner. Herewith, then, the Dr. Moser Pelvic Exam Protocol:

First, I *talk with the patient;* with pelvics, I always schedule a little extra time. I think it's important to have this conversation while the patient is still clothed. If it's the patient's first pelvic, or she has a history of problems, I approach it very differently than the pelvic given to an experienced patient – although I try to teach something during every exam. I acknowledge during this conversation that a pelvic can be an embarrassing experience.

I tell the patient what's going to happen before it happens, preparing her for sensations and sounds. I also explain each step as I do it. I offer the patient a mirror so that she can see what I'm doing.

I watch the patient's face for signs of discomfort and stop if she grimaces or looks upset – I don't believe in having her grit her teeth till it's over. I ask her to tell me when it's OK to start again, giving her control over the progress of the exam.

I stay flexible. What works for one patient might not work for another. I try to be aware of the patient's body language and tension, and be guided by her reactions.

Issues with staff. It may also happen that you become unhappy with the way you're treated by a member of the physician's staff. Do speak to your doctor about this, but be aware that she spends many hours a day with the staff and only sees you for a few minutes at a time, so mediating this kind of problem is a delicate situation. The physician will discuss the problem with the staff member, which probably will put an end to the problem. If it keeps occurring, speak to the physician again. Please don't insist that the staff member be publicly rebuked or fired.

Handling serious problems. If your health care practitioner does something really terrible – makes an overt advance to you, breaches your confidentiality, provides clearly substandard care – then it is time for direct action.

The first thing to remember under such circumstances is that you are *not* helpless. Your insurance company, your HMO, your hospital – the whole complex of people and businesses set up to take care of your health – are in the business of satisfying you. No doctor wants a reputation as someone who gives substandard care, *even* to members of sexual minorities. And if your insurance company receives several complaints about a particular practitioner, some action will follow.

So – if you are not happy with the care you are receiving, there *are* things you can do to help ensure that you'll get better care next time, and that the person who failed to take good care of you will be confronted with her error.

The first thing to do is to talk to the health care practitioner herself. Make an appointment to have this conversation, paying the copayment if she insists. Sit down with her and describe your perception of what happened, and your feelings about it: "Doctor, during our appointment last week, when I was trying to tell you about my recurring vaginal infection, you said that you thought it was sick that I had multiple sexual partners. That comment made me angry and I felt inappropriately judged. I am worried that you will not be able to provide me with good health care if you don't believe that I am mentally healthy and capable of making informed decisions about my sexual practices." Keep this conversation simple, and try not to get emotional (I know this can be hard). It may help to make a few notes beforehand about what you want to say. If you doubt your ability to remain calm having this conversation face-to-face, it's fine to call your practitioner on the phone, write her a letter, or send her an e-mail.

Once you've said your piece, give your practitioner a chance to explain her point of view. It may turn out to have been a simple misunderstanding which can be worked out so that you can go on working together.

Or it may not. If it happens that the problem is a serious one, and you don't think you can go on working with this health care practitioner, you have the absolute right to find someone else whose attitudes are more in synch with yours.

If you feel strongly that the practitioner was so out of line as to be beyond the bounds of professional behavior, you can take further action. Write a letter explaining what happened between you and the practitioner and why you are discontinuing your relationship with her. Depending on where you received your care, this letter might go to your HMO or insurance company, and/or to the Chief of Staff, Quality Assurance Department or Patient Ombudsman of the hospital or clinic where you were treated. These organizations *do* pay a great deal of attention to such input. One complaint may not trigger an investigation; however, if yours is not the first complaint they've received about this particular practitioner, you can feel sure that somebody will look into the problem.

You will not, however, get validation for your complaint – nobody will call and thank you for pointing out this doctor's inadequacies, or tell you that thanks to your letter the doctor has been dropped from their referral program. HMOs, hospitals and insurance companies do not encourage complaints; it is not in their best interests to do so. You will *not* feel empowered by the situation. However, if you feel that this is the right thing to do, your sense of helping others like you can be your motivation.

If the practitioner's behavior was really egregiously unacceptable, file a complaint with the Medical Board of your state, the governmental agency in charge of making sure that health care givers and institutions are fundamentally competent and ethical. (The address for the Federation of State Medical Boards is in the Resource Guide of this book.) Your action can help prevent harm to others.

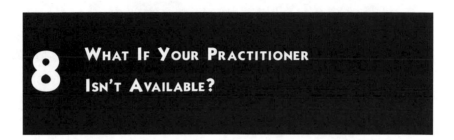

8 WHAT IF YOUR PRACTITIONER ISN'T AVAILABLE?

After all the work of finding an appropriate health care provider and coming out to him, it can be frustrating to discover that, for one reason or another, your provider is out of town or doesn't specialize in what's wrong with you or isn't on call (available) when you really need him. This situation can be particularly trying if the problem you're having is sexual in nature or is related to your sexual practices.

If your practitioner isn't around. So, here it is, Saturday night, and you need help, and your health care practitioner isn't on call. You'll have to deal with someone else, someone who may or may not have access to your medical history and who probably doesn't know anything about you or your sexual practices. The skills you practiced when you came out to your own practitioner will be helpful here.

Be respectful of the physician's time. If you reach an answering service and have to leave a message, don't place any other calls until you hear back from the practitioner – there's nothing more frustrating to a physician than receiving an urgent message and then getting a busy signal when he tries to return the call.

When you reach the physician, you'll want to take a straightforward and factual tone. Try to have a coherent story composed of relevant facts; it may help to write down key points before you place the call. Don't lie about what you were doing or leave things out – if you leave it to her imagination, she'll probably imagine something worse than what you were actually doing.

On the other hand, you don't need to explain or apologize for what you were doing, and you shouldn't spend a lot of time trying to cover all the details. Simply explain the basics of what's going on, and let the practitioner prompt you for whatever other information she needs.

You: "Hi, Dr. Strate? I'm a patient of Dr. Kool's, and I've got a problem. My partner and I were doing some bondage, and she had ropes tied around my wrists, and now my right thumb has gone numb."

Dr. Strate: "OK, I understand. How tight was the bondage? Is your hand discolored? Can you move the thumb?..." and so on.

Please don't try to play the two practitioners against one another by asking Dr. Strate to second-guess Dr. Kool, or asking Dr. Strate's opinions about the advice Dr. Kool has given you.

If you know from previous experience what kind of help you need, you can mention that to Dr. Strate. She may insist that you come in to her office, or to the emergency room, to get the problem looked at – in fact, she may have to require that you do so before she can write you certain types of prescriptions.

If what you need to help with your problem is pain medication, you will have to be fairly flexible. Health care practitioners are very restricted regarding what prescriptions they will write, particularly for a patient they haven't seen. If Dr. Strate is willing to give you a couple of doses of your medication to tide you over until Dr. Kool gets back, she is bending the rules for you, and it would be a good idea to accept with thanks. On the other hand, if she does need to see you, go on in (rereading Chapter 3, if necessary, before you go). Demanding narcotics from any doctor, much less one you've never met, is both rude and clueless.

Which brings up a tangential but important point. By getting in the habit of refilling any essential prescriptions well before you run out, you can avoid a crisis if your regular practitioner is unavailable: the person substituting for him will not have access to your medical history, and it may take several days before she can get the information she needs to authorize a refill for you. Calls like, "I need a refill of the little white football-shaped pills, I think they're for my blood pressure," are particularly frustrating: there are more kinds of little white football-shaped pills in the world than you can possibly imagine, certainly more than any doctor can remember offhand. It's also nice if you know the phone number of the pharmacy where you'd like your prescription filled.

If you need to be referred to another practitioner. Occasionally, you may have a problem that is beyond the expertise of your regular practitioner, and he will have to refer you to a specialist.

It is part of your practitioner's job to brief the new practitioner on the information she needs to do her job. If he hasn't been able to do that, or if he left out important information, you can simply give the new practitioner whatever information she needs.

You: "Hi, Dr. Gutz. Dr. Kool sent me over because I'm having some problems with my bowels."

Dr. Gutz: "Yes, I've been expecting you. Dr. Kool tells me that you have been doing anal fisting, and that you've been noticing some blood in your bowel movements. Is that correct?"

You: "Yes."

Dr. Gutz: "Is there a chance that you could have been injured by your partner's fingernail?"

You: "No, he keeps his nails filed very short and we use latex gloves"... and so on.

It's important to remember that it is not *your* job to educate the specialist; your regular physician should do that. You can act as an example your regular doctor can use for this educational process, while he ensures that you are getting the care you need. You will probably be unaware of these efforts.

It may be that you will need to be referred to a physician who may not be sympathetic to your sexual behaviors or lifestyle, but whose expertise is nevertheless needed to treat your condition. In this case you may need to ask your personal physician to act as an intermediary for you in explaining your sexuality and helping the specialist understand what he needs to know to treat you.

Once, while I was on duty in the emergency room, a transgendered person was admitted *in extremis* (near death). The on-duty anesthesiologist placed a tube in the patient's throat so that she could breathe. This anesthesiologist later made several disparaging comments about the patient to other staff members.

Well, the first thing we all did was to stabilize the patient – a life-or-death situation is no time to begin Sex Education 201. But later in the day I had a chance to talk with the anesthesiologist. I began by explaining the different types of people who fit under the heading of "transgendered." Doctors tend to be curious people, so he began to ask questions about gender and transgendered people. A half-hour discussion ensued about who transgendered people are, what they want, and what they do. I am sure this physician's views were not completely changed, but by the end of the discussion he had begun to question some of his assumptions. While I hope he will go on to learn more about all sexual and gender minorities, I believe he is today at least a little more accepting of transgendered patients. Confronting him, however, would not have helped at all, and might have further entrenched his opinions of sexual minorities. And he *did* perform the intervention that saved her life, whether he approved or not.

It would be a better world if everybody were able to listen to complaints and disagreements carefully and without defensiveness – but most of us don't live in such a world. A hostile confrontation rarely corrects a serious misunderstanding, and one experience doesn't change a lifetime of misinformation.

I know physicians who refer sexual minority patients to me, because they realize they cannot render nonjudgmental care. This is a positive step for the practitioner, not dumping. In a perfect world, they would be more willing to change their attitudes, but referring to a more understanding practitioner is a very important first step. Continuing medical education courses often do not address the issues of sexual minorities; I hope they will in the future.

If you go to the hospital. If you're checking into the hospital for an elective (that is, non-emergency) procedure, once again, it's a good idea to be straightforward and clear – most hospitals have seen it all.

If your gender presentation is ambiguous, or if your biological gender is different from your apparent gender, make that clear when you check in. The hospital may wish to arrange for a single room for you to avoid problems. Additionally, some medications and procedures vary according to gender.

Tell the hospital (usually, your admitting nurse) about any metal body jewelry that they can't see.

If you have a non-traditional family structure, it's a good idea to bring copies of any relevant paperwork such as durable powers of attorney for health care. You can also leave requests about who may and may not visit you while you're in the hospital, and who is and who is not entitled to information about your condition.

Once you're in the hospital, please act appropriately for the hospital environment, and ask your visitors to do the same. (One of my patients, admitted for an emergency appendectomy, decided that as long as his backside was hanging out of his hospital gown there was no point in wearing it at all, and had to be chased down the corridor by nurses trying to wrap a sheet around his naked body.) Your 83-year-old roommate does not need a dissertation on your love life, and your orderly probably does not want you to flirt with him. You are there to get better; relax and spend your time healing.

While it's a good idea to participate in your own health care, there's such a thing as being overinvolved. Nurses and therapists are professionals and are working under your doctor's orders; don't question everything they do. You can and should understand what they are doing to you, and asking polite questions is very appropriate: "What is this green pill?" "Why am I having an enema for wrist surgery?" It's also nice to treat them with courtesy, like the hard-working humans they are.

If you are treated rudely or unprofessionally by anyone in the hospital, it is proper to ask to see the nursing supervisor. Doing so can help protect others – sexual minority or not – from the same treatment. Most hospitals give you a patient's rights sheet on admission. Read it!

If you go to the emergency room. Once again, be straightforward. If you're in pain or scared, it can be hard to maintain a calm demeanor, but it's important to do so. Be as calm and collected as you can, and do your best to explain the problem as factually as possible. Do not demand to see a doctor right away: the nurse on duty is trained to decide which cases are more urgent, and she will get you to a doctor as soon as the next guy – the one who really will die if he isn't seen immediately – is taken care of. I assure you, the emergency room is not a popularity contest and they're not making you wait because they don't like your looks. They're not back there drinking coffee and playing cards, either – they really will help you as soon as they possibly can.

It's best, once again, to give only the amount of information needed for the nurse or doctor to understand the essential problem, and to let them ask whatever other questions they need. However, emergency room staffs see a great many cases of domestic violence and abuse, and are (rightfully) suspicious of injuries that look as though they might have resulted from abuse – so if you're marked in a way that they might think is suspicious, it's better to mention that up front.

You: "Hi, Dr. Fast. I have a laceration on my leg from where I dropped a Coke bottle and it shattered. However, I want you to know that you may also see bruises on my thigh from consensual sex play with my lover earlier this week."

If your injury resulted directly from sexual play, be upfront about explaining that. Emphasize, however, that what you were doing was consensual. It may also be a good idea to mention that you have done this before with no harm, and that what happened this time was an accident. Letting them know that your primary care practitioner is aware that you engage in these behaviors – assuming, of course, that he is – might help as well. (Do not say that your primary care practitioner "approves of" these behaviors, simply that he is aware of them.)

If you feel that anybody is giving you a hard time about your sexuality, say so: "Are you having a hard time understanding my sexuality? I think you need to learn more about this kind of sexual behavior, but right now, I'd just like you to take care of my problem."

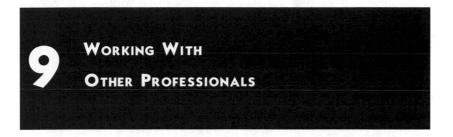

9 WORKING WITH OTHER PROFESSIONALS

For most of this book, we've been talking about interacting with physicians, chiropractors, nurses, nurse practitioners, physicians' assistants and other physical health care providers. However, doctors and the like are certainly not the only professionals with whom you might interact. There are psychotherapists, dentists, accountants, attorneys and more.

In some cases, it may not be important to come out to these professionals; it's often not directly relevant in your dealings with them, and unless it's relevant, there's no need to share information with them about your private sexual practices. On the other hand, your dentist *does* need to know that you are planning a tongue piercing while he is treating your gums, and your accountant *does* need to know about your part-time business as a professional dominant (are your corsets deductible? how about the latex?).

The time to inform your accountant that you've been depreciating your slave as personal property is *not* after you've gotten the audit notice from the IRS. Don't allow the professional to get sandbagged when something goes wrong; if there's any chance that your sexual or lifestyle practices could be relevant to the work she's doing for you, you'll have to come out to her. The information needed by the professionals you hire is determined by their need to know. Neither your physician nor your accountant needs to know that handling nickel-plated ankle fetters gives you an instant erection. Your physician may need to know about how tightly you wear them, especially considering that funny rash just on your ankles. Your accountant may need to know what you paid for them and why you think it's deductible. Your dentist would have to explain why she is asking about anklewear.

When dealing with other professionals, you will use most of the same skills and techniques we've already discussed in this book. Explain simply and straightforwardly what you do and what relevance it might have to the professional's work. If you feel like answering a few good-natured but personal questions, that's fine; if the questions seem too personal or intrusive, it's also fine to ask politely, ""How does that relate to my concerns?" Do make sure that the question-and-answer period is "off the meter" – nobody should have to pay $200/hr. for the privilege of educating their attorney or accountant.

Most professions have standards of confidentiality that are comparable to those of physicians. However, it's a bad idea to put your attorney or accountant in a position where knowing certain information can handicap him in advising you. If you are committing a crime, the professional may not be able to protect you. Since some common consensual sexual practices, such as prostitution, are crimes, ask the professional up front how much information he feels it's appropriate for you to share with him: "Mr. Counter, my sexual practices are relevant to the work we're doing together, but I'm not sure how much to tell you about them. Can you suggest some guidelines about what information to give you?"

Be clear about the difference between your personal life and your professional life. Your accountant may need information about activities that generate income; she does not need to know what you and your lovers do behind closed doors for your mutual satisfaction.

Psychotherapists. The intimate nature of the therapist/client relationship makes it very important that you find a therapist who is not judgmental about your sexuality – paying over $100 an hour to censor yourself doesn't sound like a very good deal to me.

Perhaps the most difficult task is to find a *knowledgeable* and nonjudgmental psychotherapist. Part of the therapeutic process involves being confronted with the ways in which your life is not working, despite your repeated attempts to make the same behavior patterns work. Mathematically, there are at least five possibilities:

- your problems have no relationship whatsoever to your sexuality

- your problems are the root cause of your sexual be-havior/orientation/identity, and that overcoming those problems will lead to a change in your sexuality

- your behavior/orientation/identity is the root cause of your problems, but you can learn new and better ways of expressing that sexuality which will lead to a relief of the problems

- your behavior/orientation/identity is not the root cause of your problems, but is a venue in which those prob-lems are enacted, so that overcoming the problems will lead to healthier ways of expressing your sexuality

- most likely, a mixture of the first four.

Of course, it's possible that your emotional issues might have nothing whatsoever to do with your sexuality; sometimes depression is simply depression. However, your sexuality manifests itself in many places in your life: if you're seeking help with loneliness, for example, you may even-tually want to talk to your therapist about your efforts to find friends and/or lovers – and he may not understand why you're ruling out your local church group. And a counselor who thinks any deviation from monogamy signals the end of the marriage will not understand why you and your spouse are considering an open marriage, even if both of you have agreed that it's the best way to get your special sexual needs met.

Perhaps most importantly, living in a sex-negative (sexually repressed) culture – as we all do – is an important factor in the emotional life of anybody whose sexuality doesn't fit the traditional profile of vanilla heterosexual monogamy. Remember, therapists grew up in this culture, too, and internalized many of its values. Becoming a therapist does not automatically set you free from these beliefs. If you can't trust your therapist enough to share information about your sexuality with her, how much good can you get out of your therapy?

So how do you find, and work with, a therapist who you *can* trust with the difficult stuff?

The first thing to find out is how you feel about the potential therapist as a person. Just because your friend loves her therapist doesn't mean you'll feel the same way. Interview the therapist, and ask the questions I suggested for physicians back in Chapter 2. As you listen to her answers, don't just hear the words she's saying – pay attention to her tone of voice, body language and general behavior. What sense do you get of her as a person? Does she seem intelligent and responsive? Is this someone you trust with your emotional well-being?

Next, listen to her actual words. Some therapists make sex-positive statements, but have negative feelings about particular sexualities or sexual activities – often BDSM and non-monogamy, which many therapists are still trained to see as pathological. Even if you know that this therapist is personally involved in the same sexual practices as you, that doesn't necessarily mean that she is free of judgment about that kind of sexuality – internalized oppression sneaks up on us all. Trust your instincts.

Keep in mind that you are not going to a therapist to get unconditional approval for everything you do; if that's what you want, a dog might be a better choice. Your therapist's job is to help you discover what kinds of behaviors work well for you and what kinds may be holding you back from where you want to go. If the therapist suggests to you that a particular sexual behavior or lifestyle choice may be causing certain problems in your life, that doesn't *necessarily* mean that he has negative judgments about those choices; it may actually be the case that your sexual lifestyle, or how you express it, has reached a level where it is causing significant problems in your life. On the other hand, the therapist's own conscious or unconscious beliefs about alternative sexuality may be affecting his judgment, causing him to address your sexuality as a problem when it is not.

Addressing the problem should not mean giving up your sexuality, only, perhaps, reorganizing how to make it work for you. Remember, when heterosexuals go to a therapist because their relationships are not working, the therapist does not automatically suggest they try a gay relationship.

DSM-IV (The Diagnostic and Statistical Manual, fourth edition, published by the American Psychiatric Association, which lists and defines the diagnostic criteria for all psychiatric problems) makes an important distinction in talking about non-traditional sexualities. It defines "paraphilias" as "recurrent, intense sexually arousing fantasies, sexual urges, or behaviors generally involving 1) nonhuman objects, 2) the suffering or humiliation of oneself or one's partner, or 3) children or other nonconsenting persons, that occur over a period of at least six months."

It also states that "Paraphilias must be distinguished from the *nonpathological use of sexual fantasies, behaviors, or objects as a stimulus for sexual excitement* in individuals without a paraphilia. [Emphasis mine.] ....Fantasies, behaviors, or objects are paraphiliac only when they lead to clinically significant distress or impairment (e.g., are obligatory, result in sexual dysfunction, require participation of nonconsenting individuals, lead to legal complications, interfere with social relationships." In other words, fantasies or behaviors which are consensual and which do not cause you undue distress are not paraphilias and are not pathological. Over the last several editions of the DSM, this section has become more liberal. Nevertheless, it is not the last word on the subject.

If your therapist suggests that your sexual expression is pathological, make sure he understands this section of the DSM. Many therapists seem to ignore it or have not read it.

You are seeking a therapist because parts of your life are not working. The process of fixing that problem may involve examining your entire life – the areas that you believe are working as well as those that are not. Of course, we would all like simply to remove the troubled areas without upsetting the rest of our lives; unfortunately, that is not always possible.

You're not looking for someone to "cure" you of being gay or a fetishist or polyamorous or an S/M practitioner; those things are not, in and of themselves, illnesses. (The claims of certain fundamentalist Christian groups notwithstanding, the chances of anyone being able to "cure" you are extremely slim to nonexistent anyway.) However, if your sexual desires are making it difficult for you to manage the rest of your life, or are making you unhappy, or are driving you toward doing things you find ethically unacceptable, the therapist can and should help you find more comfortable and acceptable ways to live with your sexuality.

A caveat to this permissiveness is that certain behaviors are completely unacceptable. Sex with children, in particular, is not permissible in this society. Anyone caught at, or even accused of, this behavior will experience a wide variety of severe societal sanctions. The only acceptable course of action is to work deliberately to extinguish such behaviors completely.

Be careful when a therapist suggests that all your problems arise entirely from intimacy issues, your mother, the time your babysitter touched you "there," etc. Of course, such issues can certainly be significant, but emotional difficulties are rarely so simple.

The process of therapy involves two people sitting down together, with one person a little more in touch with what is happening – usually, but not always, that person is the therapist. It is a process of forming a special relationship that can help you confront or change aspects of your feelings and behavior that are very difficult to approach alone. The therapist does not get to impose her views on you, nor does she know how you "should" be. She is not a guide, since nobody knows your destination; she is a facilitator.

At the end of therapy, you will not be ecstatically happy. Therapy is the process of trading in one set of problems for another set of problems, until you are happy with the set you have. It enables you to move past whatever problems were blocking your way prior to therapy, but will not remove all obstacles from your life forever, or even for just now.

We live in a world where we are taught that most sex is bad, and even the "right" type of sex is fraught with problems. Therapists are not insulated from these societal messages, so it can be hard to find a nonjudgmental one. Yet it can be done. If you are involved in a (real-world or on-line) community of others whose sexuality is similar to yours, try asking them first. Often, they will know of therapists who are open to people with your sexual concerns or lifestyle or behavior; if you're lucky, one or two of them will have actual experience with a particular therapist, and can tell you whether they had a good experience with her.

The Resource Guide in this book can also help guide you toward listings of therapists who consider themselves to be open to working with people of non-traditional sexualities. Some therapists advertise in gay/lesbian newspapers or in the newsletters of alternative sexuality support groups, but not all who do so are nonjudgmental.

If none of these work out for you, you'll just have to let your fingers do the walking. Most therapists should be happy to spend a few minutes with you, in person or on the telephone, so that you can get an idea of their approach and personality.

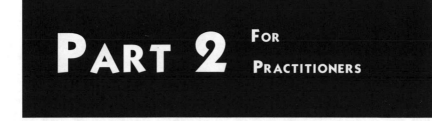

PART 2 FOR PRACTITIONERS

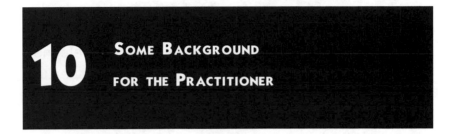

10 SOME BACKGROUND
FOR THE PRACTITIONER

(This chapter and the following chapter are adapted from two articles which first appeared in San Francisco Medicine, Nov./Dec. 1998, pp. 23-26.)

Physicians and other health care practitioners have just begun to address the special health and lifestyle issues of the gay, lesbian or bisexual patient. However, the medical concerns of other sexual minorities (including transgendered patients, patients with multiple sexual partners, sex workers, and patients involved in S/M and other "kinky" sexual behaviors) have received little to no attention. This chapter will, I hope, be a starting point for physicians and other health care professionals who wish to address the health concerns and needs of sexual minority patients.

The first question to answer for yourself is whether or not you really wish to treat such patients. Some physicians are unable to overcome their own issues about alternative sexual behaviors and should refer these patients. Even if you're a member of one sexual minority community, you may not be able to nonjudgmentally treat any or all sexual minority patients.

Just because you choose to refer these patients does not relieve you of the responsibility of learning at least the basics of how to care for them. I do not, and unfortunately never will, speak Japanese, so it is reasonable for me to refer new patients who only speak Japanese to a Japanese-speaking physician. Nevertheless, I have had to take care of such patients. I try to employ translators (both Japanese speakers who work in the hospital and family members). I have learned something of Japanese culture. The hospitals where I work have devised "Asian diets" (comfort food is important when you are sick) and have made other accommodations. Physicians confronted with sexual lifestyles with which they are not comfortable need to take similar actions: seek out experts and attempt to make accommodations for patient comfort.

If you decide that sexual minority patients will be a significant aspect of your practice, here are some recommendations on how to treat them effectively and respectfully.

Who they are vs. what they do. In treating such patients, you must distinguish between identity and behavior – a task which is not as simple as it seems. Individuals may choose to define their sexuality with a label, but their actual behavior may be very different. Medical risk is related to a patient's behavior, heredity or environment, not his or her identity. It does not matter medically whether a male patient identifies as gay, but it does matter if he has sex with men. Additionally, anal sex with a man opens him up to a different type of medical risk than anal sex with a dildo-wielding woman.

Nevertheless, identity is also an issue. A woman who self-defines as a lesbian is often subjected to a variety of stresses that a heterosexual-identified woman is not, without regard to her behavior. There are social stresses regarding partner choice ("Will my partner be allowed to visit into the MICU? What will happen when my co-workers meet my lover?"). There are also genuine physical dangers – rape, assault and even homicide – associated with being gay, lesbian, a sex worker, an S/M practitioner, or transgendered, as the crime sheet in any city can attest.

Sexual identity and behavior are both fluid. There are people who defined themselves first as gay, then straight, then bisexual. It can be hard to imagine, but there are people who are not quite sure which gender they are, people who are frustrated when no one will acknowledge their chosen gender, and people who find any gender at all intolerable. Is a woman who is happily married, but secretly desires sexual contact with other women, a lesbian or bisexual or even heterosexual? Does that orientation change if she begins an affair with another woman, if she leaves her husband, or even if she becomes celibate? There are no simple answers. Just remember that because someone identifies with one sexual orientation, it does not necessarily define their actual behavior. Acceptance of this fluidity is the first step in providing nonjudgmental health care and not alienating your patient.

Your sense of a patient's probable identity may not match up with the patient's own self-identification; you're not a mind-reader, and appearances can be deceptive. Be aware that many people, when faced with a question about someone's sexual identity, tend to categorize people into the less societally accepted roles. For example, a heterosexual man who has sex with a man is assumed to be a closeted gay, but a homosexual man who has sex with a woman is not assumed to be a closeted straight.

No assumptions. Associating certain medical problems with specific sexual minorities acts to stigmatize that minority. We all know that unprotected anal coitus is a risk factor for HIV transmission, but it may surprise some that more heterosexuals take part in anal coitus than homosexuals. The point is: talk with *all* your patients about anal safer sex practices. The assumption that you can choose whom to advise on this issue will unfortunately be proved wrong too often.

Just as an aside, anal sexuality is an area often forgotten in our medical school education. Possibly the best piece of advice you can give to patients interested in exploring anal sex is to make sure anything inserted into to the anus has a flange to prevent it from being lost in the rectum. A second safety technique, which should *also* be included, is attaching a string to the device to allow for retrieval if the flange fails to prevent the object from being lost in the rectum. Discussions of how to prevent colonic perforations (smooth soft toys, exceedingly short fingernails, quick referral for bleeding) should also be emphasized, in addition to safer sex advice. Information about sexually transmitted diseases (STDs) that can be transmitted by anal sex and oral/anal contact should also be reviewed.

How does your office appear to the sexual minority patient? Your prospective patient's first contacts with your practice are your office staff and your forms. Patient information sheets routinely ask questions that may seem simple and routine to you, but are really quite difficult. Prospective transgendered patients must choose between male and female; S/M practitioners must choose between listing their spouse or their S/M mistress as their emergency contact. How will the new doctor respond to a newly married gay couple? A new patient will judge your paperwork, before ever finding out how accepting you are.

Your office staff can be also be the cause of a misunderstanding. The odd look from your receptionist... the nurse who does not understand the need for a male doctor to have a chaperon when examining a female-to-male transsexual... the medical assistant who shudders when seeing nipple rings... the bookkeeper who refuses to explain a charge on the bill to the patient's significant other... all these can represent genuine obstacles to health care for the sexual minority patient.

The somewhat unfriendly form or staff can all lead to a hostile or fearful patient. It is probably a good idea to read over your patient materials to make sure they are not inadvertently offensive. A frank discussion with your office staff, letting them know that you welcome sexual minority patients into your practice and will not tolerate any disrespect, can also be useful. Be especially aware of the staff member who is tolerant of most sexualities, but frightened or upset by a particular sexual lifestyle or behavior; perhaps some education on your part can help allay this person's qualms.

Your own first impression. A physician who is not knowledgeable or respectful about sexual minority practices often reveals that ignorance in the initial history and physical. To avoid a bad first impression, consider some better ways of asking questions, whether you're asking them during the initial interview or on your forms:

· Rather than ask "marital status?"

Ask "Are you single, married, divorced, separated, or partnered?" The next question is "With whom do you live?"

· Rather than "What form of birth control do you use?"

Ask "Do you use birth control?" If the patient says yes, ask "What methods do you use?" If the patient says no, then ask "Do you need birth control?" (If you ask the second question first, you will overlook the patient who is relying on the rhythm method.)

· Rather than "Do you have any sexual problems?"

Ask, "Do you have any sexual concerns?" Then follow up with more detailed questions: there is research to indicate that the general question alone will not uncover sexual dysfunctions. You have to ask about each specific dysfunction: for example, do you have difficulty having an orgasm, getting an erection, maintaining an erection, with pain during sex, orgasm too soon, lubricate enough or long enough, do you desire sex? Also, referring to sexual "concerns" allows the patient to bring up concerns other than dysfunctions.

- Rather than "With how many partners do you have sex?"

  Ask, "Are you currently having sex with anyone?" If the patient says "no," you can ask "Is that a problem for you?" If the patient says "yes," you can ask "Do you have more than one partner?"

- Rather than "Who beat you up?"

  Ask, "How did you get those marks/bruises/welts?"

- Rather than "What is your sexual orientation?"

  Ask, "Do you have sex with men, women or both?"

- Finish the sex-oriented part of the interview with, "Do you engage in any sexual activities about which you have health questions?"

Respecting patients' identity and relationships. It seems only courteous to refer to patients as they request. Nevertheless, it can be difficult to remember to refer to your budding, but balding, male-to-female (MTF) transsexual patient as a "she" – to write "Frank" on the prescription, but refer to her as "Francesca." It can be hard to remember to do a pap smear on Dick, your female-to-male (FTM) transgendered patient.

I hope that you already include the patient's significant other in major decisions if that is the patient's desire, despite the relationship's legal status. Sometimes it is difficult to ferret out the relationships that are important to your patient. Your patient may have a wife and a master, or two significant others. It is appropriate and desirable to ask the patient who they would like present.

Dealing with the mistrustful patient. Many sexual minority patients mistrust traditional medicine. Some of this mistrust is understandable: many alternative sexual behaviors are also psychiatric diagnoses, and in some cases may be illegal; many patients have had less than pleasant interactions with non-accepting physicians. Reliance on alternative medicine and folk remedies, and avoidance of traditional medicine, are common. Sexual minority patients tend not to take care of health care maintenance or even simple problems. So when they finally seek medical care, there can be serious medical concerns.

For similar reasons, many sexual minority patients also mistrust mental health professionals – so a suggestion that your patient see a psychiatrist or psychotherapist may be greeted with skepticism or hostility, particularly if the patient believes that you are suggesting such therapy to "cure" the patient's sexual behavior.

I hope it goes without saying that consensual and satisfying sexual behaviors among adults that do not interfere with the patient's functioning do not need curing. Nevertheless, depression, personality disorders, stress and other psychiatric problems are at least as likely among sexual minorities as the general population. Due to the stresses of living a non-traditional lifestyle, some emotional difficulties may be more common. Illicit drug fads within (and outside) the various sexual minority communities may lead to psychiatric and medical problems. Sensitive physicians are able to assure their patients that they are recommending mental health treatment because of the psychiatric problem and not because of the sexual behavior.

Sexual minority patients are concerned, often with cause, that health care providers will pathologize them because of their sexual identity or behaviors. You will have better success with these patients if you can assure them truthfully that you do not consider their sexuality to be, in and of itself, a problem.

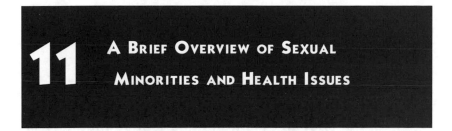

11 A Brief Overview of Sexual Minorities and Health Issues

A brief glossary of sexual minority terms. The following glossary is meant to help health care practitioners understand their patients' sexual language. It is not a complete list and not everyone will agree with these definitions, but it is a start. An accepting attitude and honest curiosity will take you a long way. Nevertheless, heed the following warnings:

1.   **Do not use these terms yourself; it is very easy to make a _faux pas_. Many of these terms can have different meanings and pejorative implications when used by someone outside the patient's sexual community; _you will be misunderstood!_**

2.   **Do not assume that someone's stated sexual orientation limits their sexual activities to within those constraints.**

3.   The definitions of these terms are seriously debated within the sexual minority communities, so these definitions are approximate and they do change over time.

4.   Even though some of these terms have pejorative meaning when used by "outsiders," they are not considered insulting when the patient uses them to self-describe or to describe friends or lovers.

5.   The italicized information in this chapter is intended to give you a very brief overview of some of the special questions and issues that may be raised during your interactions with sexual minorities. For more information, please consult the Resource Guide in the back of this book.

Sexual minorities (everything but the traditionally heterosexual) call themselves or their activities *queer, perv, pervert, kink, fetish, leather* or *leathersex.* Those who are not *sexual minorities* are called *vanilla* or *straight; vanilla* is also used to describe non-*kink* sexual activities. To be *squicked* is to be upset or disgusted by a given behavior.

Someone who is *coming out* (exploring the activity or beginning to accept the identity) is called a *novice* or *newbie.* An attractive partner is *cute* or *hot; hot* is also used to describe a particularly exciting interaction. Someone who loves *sex* (orgasm-seeking behavior) or a specific sexual activity is called a *slut.* Sometimes there is a specific type of sex that is desired, e.g., *pain slut, fuck slut,* and *anal slut.*

So many synonyms exist for male and female genitals, for breasts, and for masturbation that it is impossible to list them here. Most are in relatively common vernacular outside sexual minority communities. It is worth noting, however, that many such terms – for example, the word *cunt* – do not carry the pejorative implications in these communities that they do in the outside world.

If you're not used to this sort of language, it can be difficult not to react negatively when you hear words you've always been taught are insulting or obscene. Volunteers on one sex information support line are actually drilled on saying and hearing blunt sexual language so that they get used to it. You might consider doing something similar if language is a problem for you.

People who eroticize physical and/or psychological pain (sometimes called *intensity* or *erotic intensity*) are called *players* and are into *S/M* (aka *BDSM, sadomasochism, dominance and submission or D/S, leather,* and *bondage and discipline* or *B/D*). Some people attempt to live this as a lifestyle, *24/7* (24 hours a day, 7 days a week) or *TPE* (total power exchange). Many of these utilize *slave contracts* to spell out the rights and obligations of each partner in the relationship; although these contracts have no legal status, they often have significant moral weight. Other players only do *S/M* during sexual interactions; they do *EPE* (erotic power exchange) or *keep it in the bedroom. Players* usually adhere to the *SSC (safe, sane and consensual)* creed. A *play party* is a social gathering where *S/M* activities take place; the *party space* (venue) usually has *equipment* (large devices to which a partner can be secured). The *players* usually bring their own *toys* (handcuffs, whips, canes, etc.).

Toys are typically designed to provide sensory stimulation with minimum physical damage, and can thus help prevent many injuries. However, they can be misused. Most cities have one or more stores or organizations that teach safe use of these toys. There are also books and magazines available containing such information.

Mixed play or **cross-orientation play** implies an interaction between people who would not usually have **sex** together (a gay man with a lesbian, for example). **S/M** partners engage in **negotiation**, the process of agreeing on what will constitute the specifics of their **S/M scene** (interaction). They decide upon a **safeword** (a word or gesture that will stop the **scene**), and mutually define the **limits** (activities not to be included in the **scene**).

Players who take the active role are called **dominant, dom, domme, domina, top, master, mistress,** and **sadist. Players** who take the receptive role are called **submissive, sub, subbie, bottom, masochist, boy** or **girl,** and **slave.** (In some **S/M** interactions, it may not be immediately obvious which partner identifies as the active partner and which as the receptive partner, although the practitioner may feel strongly about the label.) **Switches** can take either role. Within the **S/M** community, there is often intense debate concerning the distinctions between these terms; it is not uncommon to hear someone say "I am a **masochist**, I will be **submissive** if my partner enjoys it, but I am no one's **slave.**"

Whipping, flogging, caning, spanking are common *S/M* activities. *Flogging* involves using a *flogger*, an instrument with several strands of leather or other material, to strike the partner. A *single-tail* is a braided implement that tapers to a narrow end. The most common place to strike is the buttocks or back, but thighs, shoulders, and genitals are also common. *Marking* (leaving bruises, welts, or generalized redness) is common, but not mandatory. Some individuals especially enjoy *play* involving a specific area of the body, e.g., *tit torture, CBT (cock and ball torture),* and *cunt torture*. *Edge play* (activities that tend to *squick* people and are more dangerous) include *blood play* (shallow piercings or cuts that draw small amounts of blood)*, knife play* (using a knife to scratch or cut, or to threaten)*, electricity* (using devices such as TENS units to deliver electrical shocks), and *breath play* or *control* (strangulation and suffocation).

These activities are not inherently abusive, criminal or self-destructive. They are typically loving, intimate and well-thought-out in terms of safety. A standard criterion for S/M play is that it should not cause damage requiring professional intervention to heal (e.g., broken bones, deep lacerations, etc.). However, even careful players sometimes have accidents. For a clearer understanding of these boundaries, it can be useful to compare S/M play to contact sports such as football or high-risk activities such as mountain climbing, and think about what kinds of injuries are commonplace, what kinds are serious but accidental, and what kinds might indicate a player who is inappropriate or out of control.

Men interested in *bears* (big, barrel-chested and usually bearded men) are called *cubs.* Men attracted to men with large penises are called **size queens**. **Daddy** and **boy** imply an **S/M** relationship; the same terms can be used by women.

Women who are interested in **sex** with other women are **lesbians** or **dykes**. **High femme** or **lipstick lesbians** are women who appear stereotypically feminine (lipstick, make-up, high heels, frilly clothes, etc.). **Femme** women may also have a decidedly feminine appearance, but not to the extreme. **Soft butch** women have a more androgynous appearance. **Stone butch** women tend to be masculine in appearance and may dislike any vaginal penetration themselves. It is common to see a **femme** woman partnered with a **butch**, but other pairings are not unusual. These roles may not be all-encompassing: some women identify with the saying "**butch** in the streets, **femme** between the sheets."

It can be tempting to try to impose the structures of typical heterosexual relationships on same-sex pairings, looking for the "man" and the "woman." While some same-sex couples identify with this paradigm, many do not, and will be extremely offended if you make assumptions regarding their roles.

Bisexuals or **bi's** are sexually attracted to both men and women. There are political forces that impel people to either embrace or deny the term **bisexual**; as one woman told me, "I have sex with both men and women, but mostly women, so that makes me a **lesbian**."

Many people engage in bisexual behavior without identifying as bisexuals. Just because your patient states that s/he is heterosexual or gay does not mean that s/he does not have sex with a gender other than his or her usual choice.

Do not assume that bisexuals are always non-monogamous; bisexuality is a matter of identity and attraction, not necessarily of behavior.

Men who like lesbians are called **dyke daddies**, but sometimes this term is used instead to mean **butches** and transgendered women interested in **daddy/boy** play. Heterosexual women who like gay men are called **fag hags** or **fruit flies**, but these terms do not usually imply sexual activity. Some lesbians interact erotically with gay men and/or in gay male environments.

Many sexual minority members like to blur the boundaries of gender: you may hear a butch lesbian refer to another butch as "he" or an effeminate man refer to a male friend as "she."

A permanent or semi-permanent marking is called a **body mod (modification)**, and is attained by tattooing (**tats**), **cuttings** (a design superficially or deeply cut into the skin by a knife or scalpel) and **piercings** (placement of metal bars or rings through the flesh). **Burns** or **burning** involve using intense heat – matches, cigars, sticks of incense – for sensation only, without attempting to create a design; they are usually thought to be temporary (healing in a matter of weeks), but can be permanent. **Branding** is the use of heat to make a permanent mark or design. Piercings have specific names for the different locations; some of the most common include **Prince Albert** or **PA** (through the frenulum and out the urethra)**, guiche** (perineum) and **triangle** (above the clitoris). Some people like the act of piercing and do **needle play** or **play piercings**, which are removed at the end of the **scene.**

Body modifications typically heal themselves within a matter of weeks or months without medical intervention. Many patients, if they encounter trouble with a body modification, will turn to the body modification artist for counsel rather than seeking medical advice. If the artist's advice doesn't work, the patient will come to you – typically with an infection that has been getting worse for quite a while. If you treat many members of sexual minorities, it might be worth while to learn more about body modifications and their ramifications, and perhaps to form affiliations with some of your local body modification studios.

A relatively common activity for both men and women is **handballing** or **fisting**, placement of a hand in the partner's anus or vagina. After the hand is inserted, it is curled into a loose fist, hence the name. Oral-anal contact is called **rimming**. A **butt plug** is a sex toy for insertion into the rectum. A **strap-on** is a **dildo** (artificial phallus), worn in a harness that allows one to engage in coitus with one's partner despite anatomy or physiology. An individual who enjoys **butt fucking** or **pumping the poop shoot** (anal coitus) is called a **back door betty** or an **anal slut. Felching** is the act of sucking one's **cum** (semen) out of a partner's rectum, and sometimes sharing it orally with the original recipient.

Not all the most "shocking" sexual activities are the most dangerous, and vice versa. If your patient trusts you enough to tell you that s/he is engaging in some of these behaviors, s/he wants and deserves nonjudgmental consultation on the possible health ramifications (HIV, Hepatitis, other STDs, as well as physical injury to the rectum or colon) of what s/he is doing. Some of these activities are not particu-

larly risky from a health standpoint, and many of the risks that do exist can be easily mitigated with latex barriers and other prophylactic strategies.

When your partner is aware that you have or could have more than one partner, you have an **open relationship.** Many people in open relationships have an **SO** (significant other) or **primary partner**, and the other relationships are called **secondary** or **fuck buddies.** Those who are open to more than one primary relationship are called **poly** or **polyamorous.** Individuals who are straightforward and honest about their activities are called **ethical sluts. Fluid-bonded** describes a relationship in which safer sex precautions are not used with that partner, but are mandatory with other partners. **Swingers** are male-female couples who seek other couples, but will occasionally allow a single to join them. The gay male version of swinging occurs at the **baths** or a **bathhouse**, which may contain **glory holes** – a hole cut in a partition through which men can engage in anonymous fellatio. Places designed for swinging or group sex are also called **sex clubs** or **sex parties**; they usually have a **group room** for group sex. **Group sex** involves orgasm seeking behavior by three or more individuals at the same time. Female-only sex parties also exist but are less common.

Non-monogamous relationships can be as healthy as any other relationship style. People in ethically non-monogamous relationships can and do maintain long-term commitments and raise happy families. The kinds of behaviors you may have encountered among the nonconsensually non-monogamous (lying, deception, etc.) are not integral to the phenomenon.

An **exhibitionist** is someone who enjoys displaying himself or herself nude, in sexy dress, or engaging in sexual behavior in front of others; a **voyeur** is someone who enjoys watching a sexual display. Both exhibitionism and voyeurism may be consensual or nonconsensual – the nonconsensual versions are illegal.

Someone can be turned on by dressing in specific garments (**drag**), which include **latex, PVC** (polyvinyl chloride), **leather**, and **corsets**. For some people, their outfit defines the fantasy that they are playing out. For the **TV** or **transvestite,** the **pony girl/boy** (someone who dresses up as a pony to pull a wagon or carry a rider), the **furrysex** aficionado (someone who role-plays being an animal having sex), or the **infantilist** (someone who role-plays being an infant), dressing up may be integral to the experience. For others it is a more comfortable way to present themselves to the world; this is not **drag**, but implies a desired life role.

A **fetish** is an erotic attraction to an inanimate object, or to a particular aspect of a human partner; some sexologists distinguish between a **fetish** (erotic attraction to an inanimate object) and a **partialism** (an erotic attraction to a body part). Common fetishes include shoes, cigars or cigarettes, and materials such as rubber or leather. Common partialisms are feet, breasts, buttocks, hair, and body fluids such as urine, blood or sweat. **Fetishwear** is costumery designed to provoke a fetishistic response, such as corsets, boots and leather motorcycle gear.

Many kinds of non-traditional erotic behaviors do not include conventional genital sexuality. Do not assume that your patient's involvement in fetishism, S/M, crossdressing or other erotic activities necessarily means that genital stimulation occurs while s/he is involved in these activities.

People who dress in the clothes of the other sex come in a variety of types: ***Transsexuals (TS)*** are people who feel that they are the other sex trapped in the wrong body. They usually desire hormonal treatment and, in some cases, gender reassignment surgery (also called sex reassignment surgery). They are often divided into ***MTF*** (male to female) or ***FTM*** (female to male) and ***pre-op*** and ***post-op*** groupings as appropriate. Transsexuals who do not intend to have surgery are called ***non-op. Transgendered (TG)*** people are those who choose not to think of themselves as one gender or the other; they may appear androgynous, or may appear as one gender at some times and another at others. Some ***TG*** people are ***TS's*** who do not desire surgery. ***Transvestites (TV)*** become sexually aroused by dressing in the clothes of the opposite sex. Most, but not all, people in this category are genetic men (although this question is debated). A ***chick with a dick*** is a ***TG*** genetic male, usually with the implication that her penis works and she will use it during ***sex;*** it can also mean a genetic woman with a ***strap-on***. A ***transsexual*** or ***transgendered*** person may refer to himself or herself as a ***T*** or a ***tranny***.

Cross-dresser is a generic term for all those who dress in the clothes of the opposite sex. ***Gender-fuck*** describes a person or activity which involves someone dressing with stereotypic aspects of both men and women at the same time (e.g., having a full beard while wearing a dress). A ***female impersonator*** or ***gender illusionist*** dresses as a woman as part of a theatrical performance. A ***drag queen*** is a gay man who dresses and acts in a stereotypically feminine style, sometimes to an outrageous and humorous extreme. A *drag king* is a lesbian who dresses and acts in a stereotypically masculine style.

Intersex or *IS* describes individuals with a biologic (genetic, physiological or anatomical) condition that produces physical aspects of both men and women. *IS* individuals may or may not consider gender an issue for them.

All these categories are extremely fluid, and one person who considers herself transgendered may dress the same, present the same way, and have the same medical issues as another who considers herself a cross-dresser or a transsexual.

Sex workers are those who earn money for providing sexual or erotic services. People who provide conventional sexual services may be *prostitutes, hookers, hustlers, whores, streetwalkers* or *callgirls. Professional dominants, pro-dommes* or *dominatrixes* provide S/M scenes in exchange for money; male professional dominants, and *pro-subs* or *professional submissives*, do exist but are rarer. *Phone sex workers*, *strippers* and *exotic dancers,* and *professional escorts* are also usually considered sex workers.

A sex worker may or may not provide conventional sexual activities such as intercourse and oral sex. S/he also may or may not use safer sex strategies. Most sex workers are at some degree of physical risk (assault, robbery, rape, homicide) and legal risk (arrest for prostitution and related crimes).

PART 3   CONCLUSION &
RESOURCE GUIDE

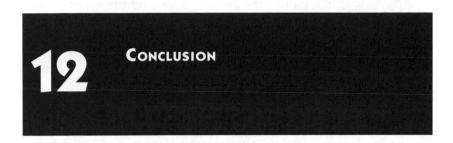

12 Conclusion

Throughout this book, I have shared my concerns about the barriers sexual minorities encounter in seeking good health care. I have recounted stories of some of the problems I've seen arise between sexual minorities and the health care system. In some cases, the problem was brought on by a health care practitioner's ignorance. In others, it was caused by the prospective patient who believed that the health care system would not or could not deliver competent treatment to someone who identifies as having an alternative sexuality.

All these problems have essentially the same solution: information. Health care professionals cannot give top-notch care to someone whose lifestyle they don't approve of or understand. Sexual minorities cannot get the health care they need if they refuse to use the system, or if they withhold information out of fear or shame.

In the incredible sexual diversity that greets us at the dawn of a new millennium, there is no excuse for ignorance. It is well past time that medical schools begin to acknowledge that patients have sex, and that this sex is often not heterosexual, marital, monogamous or "vanilla." Teaching the breadth of alternative sexualities and lifestyles should be a part of the curriculum for every mental and physical health caregiver.

With greater understanding of sex in all its diversity comes the realization that sexuality represents an enormous field for medical study and practice. Toward that end, I am establishing the American College of Sexual Medicine and Health (ACSMH). I hope that this organization of physicians interested in sexual health, the medical aspects of sexual concerns, and the sexual aspects of medical concerns, will spur the medical establishment to reach out to this underserved population. The ACSMH will work to create practice guidelines, promote research, educate physicians and other health care professionals, and identify a cadre of physicians who will be recognized by their peers for their expertise in this area of medicine. For more information about ACSMH, write to me at:

> Charles Moser, Ph.D., M.D.
> 45 Castro Street, #125
> San Francisco, CA 94114
> or check out:
> http://pweb.netcom.com/~docx2/ACSMH.html

I would like to live, and to practice medicine, in a world where quality health care is available to people of all orientations and lifestyles, and where nobody is afraid or ashamed to ask for the care they need and deserve. I hope this book will bring that world a few years closer.

> Charles Moser, Ph.D., M.D.
> April, 1999

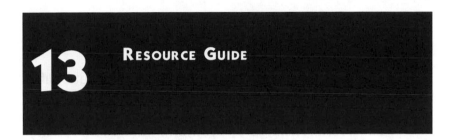

13 RESOURCE GUIDE

For help in finding a sex-positive health care pro-vider, check out the Kink-Aware Professionals list at www.bannon.com/kap. If you are a sex-positive physician, therapist or other professional, consider placing your name on this excellent resource list.

Books

Consensual Sadomasochism: How To Talk About It & How To Do It Safely. William A. Henkin, Ph.D., and Sybil Holi-day, CCSSE. Daedalus Publishing Company, San Francisco, 1996.

Loving Someone Gay. Don Clark, Ph.D. Celestial Arts, Berkeley, CA, 1997.

The Ethical Slut: A Guide to Infinite Sexual Possibilities. Dossie Easton & Catherine A. Liszt. Greenery Press, San Francisco, 1996.

The Guide to Getting It On!: A New And Mostly Wonderful Book About Sex. Paul Joannides. Goofy Foot Press, Los Angeles, 1998.

The New Joy of Gay Sex. Charles, Dr. Silverstein, Felice Picano. Harperperennial Library, 1993.

Sapphistry: The Book of Lesbian Sexuality. Pat Califia. Naiad Press, 1988.

Sex Work: Writings by Women in the Sex Industry. Edited by Frédérique Delacoste and Priscilla Alexander. Cleis Press, San Francisco, 1998.

SM 101: A Realistic Introduction. Jay Wiseman. Greenery Press, 1996.

The Transsexual's Survival Guide to Transition & Beyond. Creative Design Services, King of Prussia, PA, 1990. (Creative Design Services publishes a series of excellent pamphlets on various aspects of transsexualism. If you can't find them in the bookstore, write to them at P.O. Box 61263, King of Prussia, PA 19406.)

Magazines and Journals

for consumers:

SexLife, published by Zygote, Inc., 530 Showers Dr. #7-315, Mountain View, CA 94040, 650/968-7851. zygote@fugue.com.

for health care providers:

The Journal of Sex Research, published by the Society for the Scientific Study of Sexuality, PO Box 208, Mount Vernon IA 52314-0208. http://www.ssc.wisc.edu/ssss/jsr.htm.

The Journal of Sex Education and Therapy, published by the American Association of Sex Educators, Counselors, and Therapists, Inc. (AASECT) Suite 2-A, 103 A Avenue South, Mount Vernon, IA 52314.

Archives of Sexual Behavior, published by Kluwer Academic Publishers. (212) 620-8000. E-mail journals@plenum.com.

Organizations

The American Association of Sex Educators, Counselors and Therapists (AASECT). P.O. Box 238, Mount Vernon, IA 52314. AASECT@worldnet.att.net.

The Society for the Scientific Study of Sexuality (SSSS). P.O. Box 208, Mount Vernon, IA 52314.

Gay and Lesbian Medical Association, 459 Fulton St., Suite 107, San Francisco, CA 94102, 415-255-4547; info@glma.org.

American College of Sexual Medicine and Health. http://pweb.netcom.com/~docx2/ACSMH.html.

Sexuality Information and Education Council of the United States (SIECUS). 130 West 42nd Street, Suite 350, New York, NY 10036-7802; phone: 212/819-9770. Email: siecus@siecus.org.

In case of problems

The Federation of State Medical Boards of the United States, Inc. Federation Place, 400 Fuller Wiser Road, Ste. 300, Euless, Texas 76039-3855. (817) 868-4000. www.fsmb.org.

A listing of psychology boards nationwide can be found at http://www.psychologyinfo.com/directory/index.html.

Other Books from Greenery Press and Grass Stain Press

The Bottoming Book: Or, How To Get Terrible Things Done To You By Wonderful People
Dossie Easton & Catherine A. Liszt, illustrated by Fish $11.95

Bottom Lines: Poems of Warmth and Impact
H. Andrew Swinburne, illustrated by Donna Barr $9.95

The Compleat Spanker
Lady Green $11.95

The Ethical Slut: A Guide to Infinite Sexual Possibilities
Dossie Easton & Catherine A. Liszt $15.95

A Hand in the Bush: The Fine Art of Vaginal Fisting
Deborah Addington $11.95

Haughty Spirit
Sharon Green $11.95

Juice: Electricity for Pleasure and Pain
"Uncle Abdul" $11.95

Justice and Other Short Erotic Tales
Tammy Jo Eckhart $11.95

KinkyCrafts: 99 Do-It-Yourself S/M Toys
compiled and edited by Lady Green with Jaymes Easton $15.95

Miss Abernathy's Concise Slave Training Manual
Christina Abernathy $11.95

Murder At Roissy
John Warren $11.95

The Sexually Dominant Woman: A Workbook for Nervous Beginners
Lady Green $11.95

Sex Toy Tricks: More than 125 Ways to Accessorize Good Sex
Jay Wiseman $11.95

SM 101: A Realistic Introduction
Jay Wiseman $24.95

The Strap-On Book
A.H. Dion, illustrated by Donna Barr $11.95

Supermarket Tricks: More than 125 Ways to Improvise Good Sex
Jay Wiseman $11.95

The Topping Book: Or, Getting Good At Being Bad
Dossie Easton & Catherine A. Liszt, illustrated by Fish $11.95

Training With Miss Abernathy: A Workbook for Erotic Slaves and Their Owners
Christina Abernathy $11.95

Tricks: More than 125 Ways to Make Good Sex Better
Jay Wiseman $11.95

Tricks 2: Another 125 Ways to Make Good Sex Better
Jay Wiseman $11.95

Coming in 1999: Jay Wiseman's Erotic Bondage Handbook, by Jay Wiseman; Blood Bound: Guidance for the Responsible Vampyre, by Deborah Addington and Vincent Dior.

*Please include $3 for first book and $1 for each additional book with your order
to cover shipping and handling costs. VISA/MC accepted. Order from:*

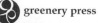 greenery press

*3739 Balboa #195 PMB, San Francisco, CA 94121
toll-free: 888/944-4434   fax: 415/242-4409   http://www.bigrock.com/~greenery*